Editorial Staff
Matthew Biagioli, MD
Wesley Smith, PhD
Sean Grieve, MS
Anthony Wyrwas, DC
Steven Wermus, MS

Book Development Staff
Paul Garbarino, MS
Tyler Poynton
B Glass Typography

Printed in the United States of America

Library of Congress Control Number: 2007926717

ISBN 978-0-9791696-1-8

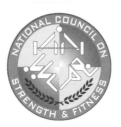

# Advanced Concepts of Personal Training Study Guide

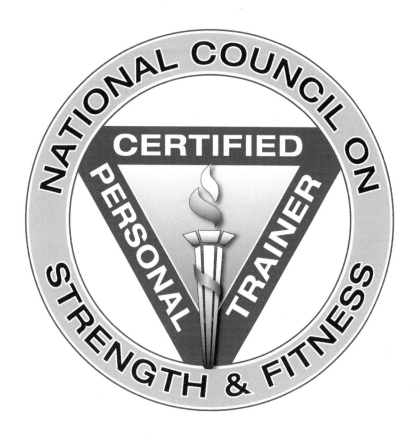

Brian D. Biagioli, EdD
Florida International University

# Table of Contents

# Lesson One
# Functional Anatomy

## Learning Objectives

- Identify the structure/composition of bones
- Identify the bones of the axial and appendicular skeleton
- Identify the major classifications of joints
- Describe the structural integrity of the different joints and the movement action associated with each joint
- Identify the gross structure and role of muscles
- Know the different movement planes of the body such as: sagittal, frontal, transverse, and the different movements taking place in each respective plane
- Know the different spatial terms such as: anterior, posterior, medial, lateral, proximal, distal, etc.
- Know the different regions of the spine and neck
- Be able to identify the different curvatures of the spine and what detrimental effects they pose to the surrounding structure
- Understand how the different anatomical positions of the pelvis are developed and how they can compromise the surrounding structure
- Be able to identify the musculature of the shoulder, shoulder girdle, elbow, wrist, trunk, hip, knee, and ankle and also be able to describe the different movement function associated with each muscle

## Match the Following Terms

1. _C_ Joint
2. _I_ Fibrous Joints
3. _k_ Cartilaginous Joints
4. _e_ Synovial Joints
5. _m_ Hyaline Cartilage
6. _o_ Fibrocartilage
7. _n_ Periosteum
8. _a_ Ligament
9. _d_ Tendon
10. _f_ Bursa
11. _b_ Muscle Fascia
12. _j_ Myofibrils
13. _l_ Myofilaments
14. _h_ Myosin
15. _g_ Actin

a) Tough fibrous band of connective tissue that supports internal organs and holds bones together properly in joints.

b) A thickened connective tissue that envelops a muscle or a group of muscles.

c) A point of articulation between two or more bones.

d) A tough band of fibrous connective tissue that connects muscles to bones.

e) Contains synovial fluid and allows for considerable movement between articulating bones.

f) A tiny fluid-filled sac that functions as a gliding surface to reduce friction between tissues of the body.

g) A protein found within the myofibril that functions with myosin to facilitate muscle contractions.

h) A contractile protein in muscle cells responsible for the elastic and contractile properties of muscle.

i) Consists of two bones that are united by fibrous tissue and exhibit little or no movement.

j) Threadlike fibrils that make up the contractile part of a striated muscle fiber.

k) Unite two bones by means of either hyaline cartilage or fibrocartilage.

l) Filaments made up of actin and myosin that are structural units of a myofibril.

m) A tough, elastic, fibrous connective tissue found in various parts of the body, such as the joints, outer ear, and larynx.

n) The dense fibrous membrane covering the surface of bones except at the joints and serving as an attachment for muscles and tendons.

o) Cartilage that allows for greater movement capabilities due to its flexible nature.

## Fill in the Blanks with Appropriate Terms

1. _Osteopenia_ refers to bone mineral density (BMD) that is lower than normal peak BMD, but not low

   enough to be classified as _Osteoporosis_, the disease state of demineralized bony tissue.

2. _Bone mineral density_ represents the mineral content of bone. The mineral content in a given volume of
   bone used

   as a measure of bony health and in the diagnosis of osteoporosis is known as the _Bone mass_.

3. The transverse cartilaginous plate near the end of a child's bone, called the _Epiphyseal plate_, is
   responsible for the lengthening growth of the bone.

4. _Hypermobility_ describes joints that stretch further than a normal range of motion.

5. A reference posture used in anatomical description in which the subject stands erect with feet parallel and arms

   adducted and supinated, with palms facing forward, is called the _Anatomical Position_.

6. _Dorsi Flexion_ is the movement of the ball of the foot toward the shin, while

   _Plantar Flexion_ represents movement at the ankle used to raise the heel from the
   ground.

7. _Abduction_ the movement away from the midline and _Adduction_ is
   the movement toward the midline of the body.

8. _External Rotation_ is the action at the shoulder and hip joint where the articulating bone is

   rotated away from the body, while _Internal Rotation_ is the action at the shoulder and hip joint
   where the articulating bone is rotated toward the body from anatomical position.

## Define the Following Terms

1. **Articular discs:** A plate or ring of fibrocartilage attached to the joint capsule + separating the articular surfaces of the bones

2. **Joint capsule:** A sac enclosing a joint is formed by an outer fibrous membrane + an inner synovial membrane.

3. **Synovial membrane:** a layer of connective tissue which lines the joint + produces synovial fluid

4. **Midline:** The median plane of the body

5. **Anterior:** Placed before or in front

6. **Posterior:** located behind a part or toward the rear of a structure

7. **Lateral:** situated or extending away from the medial plane of the body

8. **Flexion:** To bend, in hinge joints, the articulating bones move closer together, in ball + socket joints, limb moves anteriorly midline

9. **Extension:** to straighten or extend; in hinge joints the articulating bones move away from each other, in ball + socket joints, the limb moves posteriorly to midaxillary line

10. **Pronation:** Unique rotation of the forearm which crosses the radius + ulna. The palm faces posterior

11. **Supination**: Unique Rotation of forearm where the radius + ulna uncross. The palms face anteriorly

12. **Horizontal abduction**: movement away from midline

13. **Horizontal adduction**: Movement toward midline

14. **Rotation**: The turning of a structure around its long axis

## Competency Exercises

1. The organic compounds of protein, mainly in the form of collagen fiber, represent __33__ % of bone, while the mineral content represents the other __67__ %.

2. True or False?  Bone is a dynamic structure constantly undergoing changes in the body.

3. The axial skeleton consists of the __Skull__, __hyoid bone__, __vertebral column__, and __Rib cage__.

4. To promote good bone development, what three behaviors are critical?

   1. __Vitamin D__
   2. __Calcium__
   3. __Participate in Regular physical activites__

5. The three major classifications of joints are: __Fibrous__, __cartilaginous__, and __Synovial__.

6. Give an example of the synovial joint for the joint type listed.

| Joint Type | Example |
| --- | --- |
| 1. Plane Joint | 1. Spinal vertebrae |
| 2. Pivot Joint | 2. Radius/ulna |
| 3. Hinge Joint | 3. elbow + knee |
| 4. Condyloid Joint | 4. Wrist |
| 5. Saddle Joint | 5. thumb |
| 6. Ball and Socket Joint | 6. Shoulder thip |

7. The ability of the joint to move is dependent upon what 3 factors.

   1. muscular attachment location
   2. type of joint
   3. shape of the articular surface

8. True or ~~False~~? Anatomical position is the standard reference position for the body when describing locations, positions, and movements of limbs or other anatomical structures.

9. List each of the movement planes and the corresponding axis as well as two movements that occur within each plane.

| Plane | Axis | Example Movements |
|---|---|---|
| sagittal | transverse | superior to inferior / anterior to posterior |
| respective | anteroposterior | disects body front + back |
| transverse | longitudinal | splitting body into top + bottom |

10. Identify the five regions of the spine from top to bottom.

   1. (7) cervical vertebrae
   2. (12) thoracic vertebrae
   3. (5) lumbar vertebrae
   4. (1) sacral bone
   5. (1) coccygeal bone

11. ~~True~~ or False? Most disc-related injuries occur from repetitive microtrauma.

12. The primary trunk movement used for normal function is transverse flexion. What are the prime movers that support this multi-plane action?

   Trunk flexion: rectus abdominus

   Trunk rotation: spinal movements

13. Which of the following pelvic positions increases the convexity (lordosis) of the lumbar spine and may place excessive stress on the posterior aspects of the discs in the region?

        A. Neutral Pelvic Position

        B. Posterior Pelvic Tilt

        C. Anterior Pelvic Tilt

14. True or false? The glenohumeral joint is capable of movement in all planes, including hyperextension.

15. Name the four muscles that make up the rotator cuff.

    1. *supraspinatus*

    2. *infra spinatus*

    3. *teres minor*

    4. *subscapularis*

16. What upper body muscle causes both shoulder extension and shoulder adduction?
   *latissimus Dorsi*

17. The humerus is horizontally adducted by the pectoralis major, while the ___*Deltoids*___ causes horizontal abduction.

18. What muscle is used to initiate the seated row via scapular retraction?

        a. Trapezius

        b. Rhomboids

        c. Teres major

        d. Latissimus dorsi

19. In the following exercises, which hip extensor muscle is primarily responsible for the movement?

    Squat: *Gluteus maximus*

    Romanian Deadlift: *Biceps femoris*

20. Which knee muscle is also a hip flexor?

        a. vastus lateralis

        b. vastus medialis

        c. sartorius

        d. rectus femoris

*Superspinatus abducts arm*

*S*
*T*
↑
*S*

## Lesson One Quiz Questions

1.  After the age of 30, women will lose approximately what percentage of bone mass per decade?

(A) 4%
B.  8%
C.  12%
D.  14%

2.  Which of the following is an example of a hinge joint:

A.  Wrist
B.  Shoulder
C.  Neck
(D) Knee

3.  A thickened connective tissue that envelops a muscle or a group of muscles is called:

A.  Muscle fascia
B.  Myosin
C.  Myofibrils
D.  Actin

4.  Which of the following tissues connects muscle to bone?

A.  Ligaments
B.  Synovial membrane
C.  Muscle fascia
(D) Tendons

5.  Which of the following muscles is a primary hip flexor?

A.  Piriformis
(B) Gluteus maximus
C.  Psoas major
D.  Gluteus maximus

*Answers: 1 B, 2 D, 3 A, 4 D, 5 C*

# Lesson Two
# Biomechanics

- Explain Newton's three laws of physics and the different principles that support each law
- Identify the difference between internal and external force and how different forces act upon the body
- Define work, power, and the different types of energy
- Identify how torque is applied to different joints and the effects force outputs have within the body
- Explain the role of torque; how it affects movement and factors that increase it
- Define stability and identify factors that affect it
- Demonstrate a working knowledge as to the effects of gravity, rotational inertia, and angular momentum on human balance and stability
- Identify practical applications of different stabilizing units and how they affect various segments of the body
- Explain the antagonist/agonist relationship of muscle groups and their relative implications for movement economy and injury risk
- Identify proper biomechanical movements and common errors when performing the following exercises: Deadlift, Romanian deadlift, Bent-over row, Leg lifts/hip roll, Knee raise/knee rolls, Lat pull back to front, Shoulder press, Seated rows, Hip extension curl, Leg press, Supine leg curl, Leg extension, Side raise, Sit up, Triceps extension/push downs, Trunk rotation

## Match the Following Terms

1. _____ Speed
2. _____ Velocity
3. _____ Acceleration
4. _____ Energy
5. _____ Work
6. _____ Power
7. _____ Watt
8. _____ Torque
9. _____ Linear Motion
10. _____ Linear Momentum
11. _____ Kinetic Energy
12. _____ Potential Energy

a) The rate, or a measure of the rate, of motion.
b) How quickly a position changes.
c) The capacity to do work.
d) Time rate of doing work or (Force x Distance) / Time.
e) The energy possessed by a body because of its motion.
f) A change in the velocity of an object.
g) Transfer of energy by a force acting to displace a body.
h) The turning effect created by a force about an axis.
i) A unit of power in the International System of Units equal to one joule per second.
j) Energy stored by an object by virtue of its position.
k) Change in position that occurs when all points on an object move the same distance, in the same direction, and at the same time.
l) Mass of an object times the linear velocity of the object.

## Fill in the Blanks with Appropriate Terms

1. A (n)_____ load is a single sided or unbalanced load.

2. _____ is a stable state characterized by the cancellation of all forces by equal, opposing forces.

3. The distance between the fulcrum and the point of resistance is known as the _____.

4. Torque created about an axis by a pair of oppositely directed forces is referred to as _____.

5. The point where the mass of the object is equally balanced is known as the _____.

6. A group of body segments, known as a _____ ,are connected by joints so that the segments operate together to provide a wide range of motion for the limb.

7. As a rotating body spins about an external or internal axis, _____ opposes any change in the body's speed of rotation that may be caused by a torque.

8. Also thought of as "amount of rotation" of the body, _____ is the product of the momentum of a rotating body and its distance from the axis of rotation.

9. A (n) _____ refers to the role of a muscle whose torque opposes the action.

10. A (n) _____ refers to the role of a muscle whose torque aids the action, often referred to as the prime mover.

11. The force production relationship between opposing muscles or muscle groups is known as

_____.

## Competency Exercises

1. Briefly describe Newton's first three laws of motion.

   First Law: _____

   _____

   Second Law: _____

   _____

   Third Law: _____

   _____

2. Name two internal forces that act on the body.

   1. _____

   2. _____

3. Name two external forces that act on the body.

     1. _____

     2. _____

4. General motion is a combination of which two classifications of motion?

     1. _____

     2. _____

5. If the starting position is known, a particular motion can be quantified by:

     1. _____

     2. _____

6. In weightlifting, positive work is also known as a concentric contraction, while negative work is known as an eccentric contraction.
     True or False?  The body can produce more force eccentrically than concentrically.

7. Mechanical energy is held in which two forms? Give an example of each.

     1. _____   ex: _____

     2. _____   ex: _____

8. Fill in the mathematical equation for power.

     Power = _____ / _____

9. True or False?  As a muscle's contraction velocity increases, its maximal force output decreases.

10. Power output is dependent upon which two factors?

     1. _____

     2. _____

11. The torques created by the muscles of the body are dependent upon which two components?

     1. _____

     2. _____

12. Gravity pulls on the center of mass of an object at the rate of _____ m/sec$^2$.

13. List three variables that can be manipulated to achieve bodily stability.

    1. _____

    2. _____

    3. _____

14. Name the four components that make up the inner unit of the lumbopelvic region.

    1. _____

    2. _____

    3. _____

    4. _____

15. The _____ represents the primary stabilizer for the lumbopelvic region.

16. The amount of rotational inertia produced is dependent upon which three factors?

    1. _____

    2. _____

    3. _____

17. For each of the following lifts give one common error observed when performing the lift, the potential harm the incorrect movement could pose, and the method for correcting the particular movement error.

    1. **Deadlift**:

    Error: _____

    _____

    Potential harm: _____

    _____

    Correction: _____

    _____

2. **Leg lifts to hip rolls**:

   Error: _____

   _____

   Potential harm: _____

   _____

   Correction: _____

   _____

3. **Lat pull-down**:

   Error: _____

   _____

   Potential harm: _____

   _____

   Correction: _____

   _____

4. **Leg press**:

   Error: _____

   _____

   Potential harm: _____

   _____

   Correction: _____

   _____

5. **Sit up**:

   Error: _____

   _____

   Potential harm: _____

   _____

   Correction: _____

   _____

## Lesson Two Quiz Questions

1. When swimming, water is an example of what type of resistive force?

    A. Tensile force
    B. Compressive force
    C. Non-Contact force
    D. Contact force

2. The concentric phase of a military press is an example of which of the following?

    A. Negative work
    B. Positive work
    C. Potential energy
    D. Frictional force

3. Which of the following has the greatest effect on a measured power output?

    A. Muscle initial length
    B. Neutralizing properties
    C. Contractile velocity
    D. Location of the center of gravity

4. Leg lifts are contraindicated due to:

    A. The resistive torques place excessive stress on the rectus abdominis
    B. The cervical spine may become strained
    C. The hip flexors cause anterior pull on the spine leading to disc compression
    D. The pelvis is pulled into a posterior tilt

5. What is a common biomechanical problem caused by performing the leg press exercise with tight hip extensors?

    A. Pelvis migrates into a posterior pelvic tilt
    B. The knees are forced past the toes
    C. Cervical spine stress occurs due to neck flexion
    D. All of the above

*Answers 1 D, 2 B, 3 C, 4 C, 5 A*

# Lesson Three
# Muscle Physiology

## Learning Objectives

- Identify the different muscle tissue types and characteristics that differentiate them
- Identify muscle structure/composition and the pathways involved in muscle contraction
- Explain the factors that affect force production capabilities within the muscle tissue
- Explain the role of muscle spindles and Golgi tendon organs
- Discuss the different factors that contribute to short-term and long-term muscle fatigue and recovery rate
- Define the different types of muscle contractions and explain how they are used in human movement
- Compare and contrast the metabolic characteristics of the different muscle fibers and explain their role in force production under varying intensities and speeds
- Explain how muscle fiber distribution affects training outcomes

## Match the Following Terms

1. _h_ Skeletal Muscle

2. _B_ Cardiac Muscle

3. _m_ Smooth Muscle

4. _a_ Sarcolemma

5. _I_ Endomysium

6. _C_ Motor Unit

7. _J_ Concentric contraction

8. _d_ Eccentric contraction

9. _e_ Isometric contraction

10. _g_ Type IIb fibers

11. _l_ Type IIa fibers

12. _k_ Type I fibers

13. _f_ Myoglobin

a) A thin polarized membrane enclosing a striated muscle fiber.

b) A type of involuntary, mononucleated, or uninucleated, striated muscle found exclusively within the heart.

c) A motor neuron and all of the corresponding muscle fibers it innervates.

d) A type of muscle contraction in which the resistance is greater than the force applied by the muscle so that the muscle lengthens as it produces force.

e) A contraction in which muscle tension is increased, but the muscle is not shortened because the resistance cannot be overcome. There is no change in muscle length or joint angle.

f) The oxygen-transporting protein of muscle, resembling blood hemoglobin in function.

g) A large-diameter muscle fiber characterized by a reliance on the glycolytic pathways. This fiber type is quick to fatigue but is capable of high power outputs.

h) A type of striated muscle attached to the skeleton and used to facilitate movement, by applying force to bones and joints via contractions.

i) The fine connective tissue sheath surrounding a muscle fiber.

j) A type of muscle contraction in which the muscle applies accelerating force to overcome the resistance. The length of the muscle shortens as force is produced.

k) A small-diameter muscle fiber characterized by aerobic metabolism and lower maximum tension. This fiber type is fatigue resistant and highly oxidative.

l) An intermediate-diameter muscle fiber characterized by aerobic and anaerobic metabolism.

m) A type of non-striated muscle found within the "walls" of hollow organs.

## Fill in the Blanks with Appropriate Terms

1.  Tiny blood vessels called ___capillaries___ network throughout the body, passing oxygen and nutrients into tissue cells.

2.  ___Troponin___ is a protein complex found in both skeletal muscle and cardiac muscle that relays calcium sensitivity to muscle cells; while ___Tropomyosin___ binds to molecules of actin and troponin to regulate the interaction of actin and myosin.

3.  _____ is used to fuel mechanical work.

4.  Specialized muscle structures called ___Muscle spindles___ innervated by both sensory and motor neuron axons, functioning to send proprioceptive information about the muscle to the central nervous system, in response to muscle tissue length.

5.  Kinesthetic receptors called ___Golgi tendon organs___ are situated near the junction of muscle fibers and a tendon and act as muscle-tension regulators.

## Competency Exercises

1.  Identify the muscle tissue based on the description of that muscle type.

    1.  Comprises the muscular walls of blood vessels as well as the gastrointestinal tract.
        1.  ___smooth___

    2.  Located in the heart
        2.  ___cardiac___

    3.  Acts on the skeleton to maintain posture, create voluntary movement, and manage force transfer.
        3.  ___skeletal___

2.  A muscle fiber is either in a state of producing maximum tension or not producing any tension at all, which is termed _____.

3.  List 3 ways in which the neuromuscular system will increase the force production of the muscle tissue.

    1.  _____

    2.  _____

    3.  _____

4.  Name the three muscle fiber contractions.

1. _twitch_

2. _Sustained muscle contractions_

3. _complete tetanus_

5.  List five causes of short-term muscle fatigue.

1. _exhaustion of ATP/CP reserves_

2. _Decreased muscle PH_

3. _Insufficient oxygen_

4. _Reduced enzyme activity_

5. _Tubular system disturbance_

6.  List the three causes of long-term muscle fatigue.

1. _Depleted glycogen + blood glucose levels_

2. _Damage to sarcoplasmic reticulum_

3. _Depletion of electrolyte ions_

7. Name the fiber types (type I, type IIa, type IIb) based on their metabolic characteristic descriptions.

1.  Fast Fatigue/Fast Twitch,
    High power output,
    Large fiber diameter.

1. _Type IIb_

2.  Fatigue Resistant/Slow Twitch,
    Low power output,
    Small fiber diameter.

2. _Type I_

3.  Fatigue Resistant/Fast Twitch,
    Intermediate power output,
    Intermediate fiber diameter.

3. _Type IIa_

8. True or False?  Fast twitch muscle fibers preferentially function using the anaerobic metabolic systems, while slow twitch muscle fibers are more efficient in the aerobic metabolic system.

9. True or False? Information regarding recruitment and fiber characteristics is not relevant when creating the exercise prescription.

## Lesson Three Quiz Questions

1.  Which of the following muscle types maintains the highest concentration of mitochondria?

    A.  Smooth Muscle
    B.  Skeletal Muscle
    C.  Cardiac Muscle
    D.  All of the above

2.  Exercise-related fatigue may occur in _____ compromising performance.

    A.  The central nervous system
    B.  The peripheral nervous system
    C.  The muscle fiber
    D.  All of the above

3.  What type of muscle contraction is commonly used for stabilization and is characterized by no change in the joint angle?

    A.  Isometric contraction
    B.  Eccentric contraction
    C.  Concentric contraction
    D.  All of the above

4.  Which of the following is a kinesthetic receptor situated near the junction of muscle fibers and a tendon which serve as muscle-tension regulators?

    A.  Mitochondria
    B.  Sarcolemma
    C.  Muscle spindles
    D.  Golgi tendon organs

5.  Which muscle fiber type would be the most predominant contributor to performance for an endurance athlete?

    A.  Type I fibers
    B.  Type IIa fibers
    C.  Type IIb fibers
    D.  None of the above

*Answers 1 C, 2 D, 3 A, 4 D, 5 A*

## Lesson Four
## Endocrine System

### Learning Objectives

- Discuss the four general categories of hormone actions
- Identify the different endocrine glands and the hormones each gland produces
- Discuss the interrelationship between exercise, psychological/physiological stress, and immune function
- Explain how stress affects the adrenal hormone and the consequences associated with a chronic response
- Explain the role of anabolic hormones in muscle hypertrophy
- Describe factors that affect the hormonal response to resistance training
- Explain the general hormone response to endurance training

## Match the Following Terms

1. _____ Eustress

2. _____ Distress

3. _____ Steroid

4. _____ Lipid

5. _____ Ribosomes

6. _____ DHEA

7. _____ Androstenediol

8. _____ Androstenedione

9. _____ Gynecomastia

10. _____ Catecholamines

11. _____ Adrenocortical hormone

12. _____ Insulin

13. _____ Glucagon

a) A natural steroid hormone produced from cholesterol by the adrenal glands.

b) A group of organic molecules that includes fats, oils, and waxes.

c) Any naturally occurring amine functioning as a neurotransmitter or hormone.

d) Small particles, present in large numbers in every living cell, whose function is to convert stored genetic information into protein molecules.

e) A positive, desirable form of stress that influences physical or physiological health.

f) An unsaturated androgenic steroid that has a weaker biological potency than testosterone.

g) Any of a group of organic compounds belonging to the general class of biochemicals called lipids, which are easily soluble in organic solvents and slightly soluble in water.

h) A negative form of stress that influences physical or physiological health.

i) An unsaturated steroidal derivative of androstane.

j) Any of the various hormones secreted by the adrenal cortex.

k) Overdevelopment of the mammary glands in males; male breast development.

l) A hormone produced by the pancreas that stimulates an increase in blood sugar levels.

m) A natural hormone made by the pancreas that controls the level of the sugar glucose in the blood.

## Define the Following Terms

1. **Endocrine system**:

2. **Homeostasis**:

3. **Hormone receptors**:

4. **Target cell specificity**:

5. **Polypeptides**:

6. **Hypertrophy**:

7. **Androgenic hormone**:

## Competency Exercises

1. The primary endocrine glands include the:

      1. _____

      2. _____

      3. _____

      4. _____

      5. _____

2. Hormonal activity will generally fall under one of four categories including:

      1. _____

      2. _____

      3. _____

      4. _____

3. Hormones are categorized into two classes:

      1. _____

      2. _____

4.  Name four stressors that have a negative impact on immune function.

    1. _____

    2. _____

    3. _____

    4. _____

5.  Fill in the appropriate box with either a(n) Endocrine Gland, Hormone, or Action.

| Endocrine Gland | Hormone | Action |
|---|---|---|
|  | Growth Hormone | Stimulates IGF, protein synthesis, growth, and metabolism |
| Thyroid | Thyroxine |  |
| Adrenal Cortex |  | Promotes use of fatty acids and protein catabolism; conserves sugar; maintains blood glucose level<br><br>Promotes sodium, potassium metabolism and water retention |
|  | Epinephrine<br><br>Norepinephrine |  |
|  | Insulin<br><br>Glucagon | Promote glucose uptake by the cell, stores glycogen; aids in protein synthesis<br><br>Releases glycogen from the liver to increase blood glucose concentrations |
| Liver |  | Increases protein synthesis |
| Ovaries | Estrogen |  |
|  | Testosterone |  |

6. Name five hormones that contribute to anabolic activity.

1. _____

2. _____

3. _____

4. _____

5. _____

7. The concentration of testosterone in women is _____ times less than in men.

    A.  5
    B.  10
    C.  15
    D.  20

8. For optimal fat utilization and a reduced risk of fat storage caused by high blood glucose concentrations, dietary

    intake of excess _____ and

    _____ should be controlled to reduce the effects of insulin.

9. Triiodothyroxine aids in the development of lean mass by stimulating an increased secretion of which two hormones?

    1. _____

    2. _____

10. The adrenal glands produce two categories of hormones referred to as:

    1. _____

    2. _____

11. True or False? The tissues become more resourceful as disruptive environments force them to improve in efficiency.

12. The specific response by the working tissues and the endocrine glands that mediate their action is dictated by:

    1. _____

    2. _____

13. True or False?  Type II muscle fibers experience a far more dramatic effect in protein synthesis than type I fibers.

14. Place a directional arrow for the effect the type of training, either resistance or endurance training, will have on a particular hormone (↑ increase, ↓ decrease, or ↔ no change).

| Resistance Training | Endurance Training |
| --- | --- |
| _____Growth hormone | _____Growth hormone |
| _____Testosterone | _____Testosterone ( as intensity increases ) |
| _____Insulin | _____Insulin |
| _____Thyroxine and Triiodothyronine | _____Thyroxine and Triiodothyronine |
| _____IGF | _____IGF |
| _____Cortisol ( in heavy exercise only ) | _____Cortisol (related to available energy and duration) |
| _____Epinephrine ( in heavy exercise ) | _____Epinephrine (increases with intensity) |

15. Name three common errors in bodybuilding or activities aimed at muscle hypertrophy.

1. _____

2. _____

3. _____

# Lesson Four Quiz Questions

1.  Growth hormone (GH) is excreted by which of the following endocrine glands?

    A.  Thyroid
    B.  Testes
    C.  Adrenal Medulla
    D.  Anterior Pituitary


2.  All of the following are reasons cortisol is viewed as a catabolic hormone except:

    A.  It increases proteolytic enzymes
    B.  It converts amino acids to glucose
    C.  It decreases muscle cell degradation
    D.  It inhibits protein synthesis


3.  Protein enhancements leading to greater size and strength of the tissue as a result of cellular stimulation and hormone interaction take place in the _____.

    A.  Actin
    B.  Myosin
    C.  Structural non-contractile proteins
    D.  All of the above


4.  The production of which of the following anabolic hormones is reduced in response to an acute bout of resistance training?

    A.  Insulin
    B.  Testosterone
    C.  Growth Hormone
    D.  Insulin-like Growth Factor


5.  What rest interval is associated with the greatest anabolic hormone response to resistance training when the exercise is performed for 8-12 repetitions using 70%-80% of 1RM?

    A.  30-60 seconds
    B.  60-120 seconds
    C.  120-180 seconds
    D.  The rest interval does not affect the hormone response


*Answers 1 D, 2 C, 3 D, 4 A, 5 A*

# Lesson Five
# Bioenergetics

## Learning Objectives

- List the caloric density of protein, carbohydrates, fat, and alcohol
- Explain the time: intensity relationship of energy utilization during anaerobic exercise
- Discuss how the metabolic pathway affects exercise program decisions
- Describe the means by which ATP is supplied to the muscle during the transition from rest to steady-state work
- Explain the process of ATP/CP rephosphorylation and identify the relative duration for complete replenishment following a maximal effort
- Discuss how the byproducts of glycolysis may inhibit force production
- Identify the storage locations for sugar in the body and explain how glycogen utilization affects fatigue
- Explain how lactic acid is utilized by the body
- Compare and contrast the formation of ATP through aerobic and anaerobic means and how the metabolic pathway affects force production
- Identify the components in muscle tissue that contribute to the aerobic process
- Explain how lipids and proteins are used as a fuel for activity
- Discuss the different types of fatigue and how they occur in response to exercise
- Explain how excess macronutrients are stored as lipids

## Match the Following Terms

1. _____ Calorie

2. _____ Kilocalorie

3. _____ Enzyme

4. _____ Creatine Phosphate

5. _____ Creatine Kinase

6. _____ Mitochondria

7. _____ Lactic Acid

8. _____ Pyruvate

9. _____ Lactate

10. _____ Triglycerides

11. _____ Albumin

12. _____ Lipoproteins

13. _____ Amino Acids

14. _____ Central Fatigue

a) An energy substrate produced during the metabolic breakdown of glucose.

b) Consists of a glycerol and three fatty acids bound together in a single large molecule; an important energy source forming much of the fat stored in the body.

c) Basic organic molecules consisting of hydrogen, carbon, oxygen, and nitrogen that combine to form proteins.

d) Compounds of protein that carry fats and fat-like substances such as cholesterol in the blood.

e) A blood protein produced in the liver that helps to regulate water distribution in the body.

f) An energy substrate deemed as the end-product in glycolysis.

g) A unit measuring the energy value of foods.

h) A protein that catalyzes a biochemical reaction or change.

i) A unit of energy equal to the amount of heat required to raise the temperature of one kilogram of water by one degree Celsius at one atmospheric pressure.

j) An intracellular organelle responsible for generating most of the ATP required for cellular operations.

k) The buffered form of lactic acid which can serve as an additional energy source.

l) An organic compound found in muscle tissue and capable of providing rapid energy for muscular contractions.

m) An enzyme present in muscle and other tissues that catalyzes the reversible conversion of ADP and phosphocreatine into ATP and creatine.

n) The component to fatigue generally described as a reduction in the neural drive or nerve-based motor command to working muscles which results in a decline in the force output.

## Fill in the Blanks with Appropriate Terms

1.  In the absence of freely available oxygen, the process of energy production in the body is known as

    _____.

2.  The metabolic process called _____ breaks down carbohydrates and sugars through a series of reactions to either pyruvic acid or lactic acid and releases energy for the body in the form of ATP.

3.  _____ is the process of generating glucose from other organic molecules like pyruvate, lactate, glycerol, and amino acids to fuel exercise and physiological energy demands.

4.  The difference between oxygen uptake of the body at the onset of exercise and when it reaches a steady-state is

    known as _____.

5.  _____ is the term used to describe the amount of extra oxygen required by muscle tissue during recovery from vigorous exercise.

6.  _____ is an enzyme capable of breaking down a lipid in a process known as

    _____.

7.  When a fatty acid is not attached to other molecules it is known as a _____.

8.  _____ is the process by which fats are broken down in the mitochondria to generate Acetyl-CoA, the entry molecule for the Citric Acid Cycle.

9.  A series of oxidation-reduction reactions called the _____ take place during the aerobic production of ATP.

## Competency Exercises

1.  Identify the number of calories per gram as established by the Atwater general factors for the following.

    | | |
    |---|---|
    | Proteins | _____ |
    | Fats | _____ |
    | Carbohydrates | _____ |
    | Alcohol | _____ |

2.  The body uses its stored ATP during a single, maximal effort exercise in about 1-3 seconds and requires at least _____ seconds to fully replenish its stores.

3.  _____ is used as a secondary immediate fuel source, which releases energy

    when split by the enzyme _____ and can fuel reactions lasting 10-15 seconds but

    takes between _____ minutes to restore.

4.  The product of glycolysis is two molecules of _____ and two energy substrates,

    _____ or _____ .

5.  Anaerobic exercise intensities between _____% & _____% should be employed to volitional failure to
    effectively challenge the glycolytic energy system.

6.  What is the predominant energy pathway for maximal biological work lasting up to 3 minutes?

    _____

7.  What is the Krebs cycle and what is the end product?

    _____

    _____

    _____

8.  What are the three largest determinants of efficiency during aerobic exercise?

    1. _____

    2. _____

    3. _____

9.  Amino acids can be turned into what two things before entering the Krebs cycle?

    1. _____

    2. _____

10. When lactic acid accumulation is high enough to drop the blood's pH level down to 6.8 from a normal 7.4,
    physical exhaustion ensues, resulting in what negative side effects?

    1. _____

    2. _____

    3. _____

    4. _____

11. True or False? Glycogen uptake is promoted immediately following exercise.

## Lesson Five Quiz Questions

1. What type of acid is associated with a burning sensation in active tissue during high intensity exercise?

   A. Fatty acids
   B. Citric acid
   C. Lactic acid
   D. Amino acids

2. High intensity anaerobic exercise may be limited by contractility inhibition due to the presence of which of the following?

   A. Hydrogen ions
   B. Nitrogen
   C. Carbon dioxide
   D. All of the above

3. Improved glucose-sparing associated with endurance training enhances the ability of the muscle to use which of the following fuel sources?

   A. Proteins
   B. Lipids
   C. Amino acids
   D. Carbohydrates

4. Even with sufficient levels of oxygen and lipids to meet the intensity demands of work, significant fatigue will ensue when _____ becomes depleted.

   A. Carbohydrates
   B. Proteins
   C. Amino acids
   D. Creatine

5. What is the primary energy source used to fuel a 3RM squat performance?

   A. Stored ATP
   B. Creatine Phosphate
   C. Glycogen
   D. Lactate

6. For optimal performance, what is the minimal rest interval between tests for vertical jump based on proper ATP replenishment?

   A. 30 seconds
   B. 90 seconds
   C. 120 seconds
   D. 3 minutes

*Answers  1 C, 2 A, 3 B, 4 A, 5 B, 6 B*

# Lesson Six
# Cardiovascular Physiology

## Learning Objectives

- Identify the different chambers and valves of the heart and explain how they interact to maintain proper blood flow
- Describe the path of blood flow through the heart
- Explain how heart rate is regulated
- Identify the mechanism for oxygen transport in the blood
- Explain why cardiac tissue is specialized for nonstop contractility
- Define and calculate cardiac output
- Discuss how blood pressure is regulated and identify variables that affect its value
- Develop a basic understanding of the network of arterial and venous blood flow throughout the body
- Explain how oxygen and nutrients are exchanged in tissues of the body
- Identify palpation sites and measure a person's pulse at the carotid and radial arteries
- Identify the mechanisms for regulating blood flow and blood pressure response during exercise
- Describe the ventilation mechanisms involved in regulating oxygen requirements in response to the demands of exercise

## Match the Following Terms

1. _____ Atria

2. _____ Ventricle

3. _____ Superior vena cava

4. _____ Tricuspid valve

5. _____ Pulmonary semilunar valve

6. _____ Pulmonary vein

7. _____ Bicuspid valve

8. _____ Aortic semilunar valve

9. _____ Aorta

10. _____ Sinoatrial (SA) node

11. _____ Atrioventricular (AV) node

12. _____ Conducting arteries

13. _____ Arterioles

14. _____ Veins

a) A small mass of specialized cardiac muscle fibers that controls the heartbeat.

b) A valve of the heart, composed of two triangular flaps, that is located between the left atrium and left ventricle, serving to regulate blood flow between these chambers.

c) The major artery that carries oxygenated blood from the heart, to be delivered by arteries, throughout the body.

d) The two lower chambers of the heart, which receive blood from the atria and pump it either to the lungs or the body.

e) Deliver large quantities of blood to different regions of the body.

f) A blood vessel that returns deoxygenated blood to the heart.

g) The two upper chambers of the heart, which receive deoxygenated blood from the veins and oxygenated blood from the lungs and push it into the ventricles.

h) A semilunar valve between the right ventricle and the pulmonary artery; prevents blood from flowing from the artery back into the heart.

i) The primary vein collecting blood from the head, chest wall, and upper extremities and draining into the right atrium.

j) A three-segmented valve of the heart that keeps blood in the right ventricle from flowing back into the right atrium.

k) One of the small, thin-walled arteries that end in capillaries.

l) A small mass of specialized cardiac muscle fibers between the atria and the ventricles of the heart, which conducts the normal electrical impulse from the atria to the ventricles.

m) A vein that carries oxygenated blood from the lungs to the left atrium of the heart.

n) A heart valve comprising three flaps which guard the passage from the left ventricle to the aorta and prevents the backward flow of the blood.

## Fill in the Blanks with Appropriate Terms

1. _____ is the contraction of the chambers of the heart to drive blood into the aorta,

   while _____ is the relaxation and dilation of the heart chambers during which
   time they are filled.

2. Part of the impulse-conducting network of the heart, called _____, rapidly
   transmit impulses from the atrioventricular node to the ventricles.

3. The _____ is the electrical activation of the myocardium that occurs in the
   sinoatrial (SA) node.

4. The _____ is the volume of blood pumped out of the left ventricle of the
   heart in a single beat.

5. The _____ is the number of heartbeats per unit of time, usually
   expressed as beats per minute.

6. _____ is the volume of blood being pumped by the heart per
   unit of time. It is equal to the heart rate multiplied by the stroke volume.

7. The pressure exerted by the blood against the walls of the blood vessels is known as

   _____.

8. _____ is a chronic condition characterized by thickening and hardening

   of the arteries and a build up of plaque on arterial walls, while _____ is a
   stage of arteriosclerosis, in which the arteries become clogged by the build-up of fatty substances.

9. _____ is a form of low blood pressure often precipitated by
   moving from a lying or sitting position to standing up straight.

10. The _____ maneuver is a strain against a closed airway
    combined with muscle tightening, such as when a person holds his or her breath and tries to exert a significant
    force.

## Define the Following Terms

1. **Hemoglobin**:

2. **Bicarbonate**:

3. **Alveoli**:

4. **Myocardium**:

5. **Plaque**:

6. **Venules**:

7. **Blood pooling**:

8. **Plasma**:

9.  **Red blood cells**:

10. **White blood cells**:

11. **Platelets**:

12. **Hematocrit**:

13. **Coronary circulation**:

14. **Rate pressure product**:

## Competency Exercises

1. Name the four chambers of the heart.

    1. _____

    2. _____

    3. _____

    4. _____

2.  Give the route de-oxygenated blood travels, beginning with how it returns to the heart.

    1. Right atrium _____ ; to the,

    2. Right ventricle _____ ; to the,

    3. Pulmonary artery _____ ; to the,

    4. Pulmonary vein _____ ; to the,

    5. left atrium _____ ; to the,

    6. left ventricle _____ ; to the,

    7. Aorta _____ .

3. What is the function for each of the following heart valves?

    1. Tricuspid valve - _____.

    2. Pulmonary semilunar valve - _____.

    3. Bicuspid valve - _____.

    4. Aortic semilunar valve - _____.

4. The two nodes responsible for dictating the contractile element of the heart via electrical signals are known as:

       1. _____

       2. _____

5. Define the following terms.

      Stroke Volume - _____

      Heart Rate - _____

      Cardiac Output - _____

6. Cardiac Output = _____ X _____

7. Give three negative side effects of blood pooling.

       1. _____

       2. _____

       3. _____

8. Name the most commonly palpated artery at each of the following locations.

      Neck              _____

      Arm                _____

      Upper Arm       _____

      Leg                _____

9. Name four components or behaviors that increase the risk for arteriosclerosis.

       1. _____

       2. _____

       3. _____

       4. _____

10. Due to their reduced efficiency at regulating blood pressures, personal trainers should be cautious when working with what two populations?

    1. _____

    2. _____

11. True or False? Most varicose veins are not a serious medical problem, but they sometimes can lead to complications.

12. List six ways in which blood functions within the body.

    1. _____

    2. _____

    3. _____

    4. _____

    5. _____

    6. _____

13. There are _____ liters of blood in the body.

    A. 0-1
    B. 2-3
    C. 4-5
    D. 6-7

14. Blood flow to the tissues is regulated by what three mechanisms?

    1. _____

    2. _____

    3. _____

15. Name five factors that increase blood pressure during resistance training exercises.

    1. _____

    2. _____

    3. _____

    4. _____

    5. _____

16. During an exercise bout, ventilation will be controlled by:

    1. _____

    2. _____

    3. _____

17. An improved rate of _____ extraction from the blood occurs in response to

_____ adaptations.

## Lesson Six Quiz Questions

1. The hardening of the arteries associated with the cascade of events that lead to vessel blockage is called
   _____.

   A. Arteriosclerosis
   B. Orthostatic hypotension
   C. Hyperlipidemia
   D. Hypertension

2. Which of the following cardiovascular aspects increases in response to a greater cardiac output associated with exercise?

   A. Diastolic blood pressure
   B. Systolic blood pressure
   C. Vasoconstriction
   D. Blood pooling

3. Which of the following are tiny vessels where oxygen and nutrients diffuse into the cells?

   A. Arteries
   B. Veins
   C. Capillaries
   D. Mitochondria

4. Approximately what percentage of the blood is located in venous circulation?

   A. 20%
   B. 40%
   C. 65%
   D. 85%

5. Which artery is palpated when taking a pulse at the neck?

   A. Temporal artery
   B. Brachial artery
   C. Carotid artery
   D. Femoral artery

*Answers: 1 A, 2 B, 3 C, 4 C, 5 C*

# Lesson Seven
# Nutrition: Energy Yielding Nutrients

## Learning Objectives

- List the six classes of nutrients
- Identify the components of an energy yielding nutrient
- Differentiate the categories of carbohydrates and explain their relative characteristics
- List the benefits and role of fiber in a diet and identify food sources high in fiber content
- Explain the relationship of sugar and glycemic response and the risks of a high sugar diet
- Define glycemic index and glycemic load and explain their relationship with blood glucose
- Discuss possible consequences of eating a diet rich in processed carbohydrates
- Identify the risks and understand the physiological consequences of dieting with carbohydrate restriction
- Explain the relevance of maintaining stable blood glucose levels
- Define hunger and appetite
- Discuss the relationship of carbohydrates to protein-sparing mechanism
- Explain the relationship of carbohydrate intake and exercise performance
- Calculate carbohydrate intake requirement
- List the three categories of lipids
- Identify the role of fats/lipids in a diet
- Compare and contrast saturated and unsaturated fat in the diet
- Identify dietary fat sources that present possible risk for disease when over-consumed in the diet
- Explain the relationship between saturated fat and blood cholesterol
- Define hydrogenation and explain the effects of Trans-fatty acids in the diet
- Know the recommended requirements of fat in a healthy diet and the consequential effects of high fat diets
- Define the term essential nutrient
- Explain the difference between complete and incomplete proteins
- Describe key functions of protein and factors that affect the daily requirements
- Identify the highest recommended intake of protein in the diet and the negative consequences associated with excessive protein consumption

---

## Define the Following Terms

1. **Soluble Fiber Sources**:

2. **Insoluble Fiber Sources**:

3. **Glycemic Response**:

4. **Glycemic Load**:

5. **Hunger Mechanism**:

6. **Compound Lipids**:

7. **Derived Lipids**:

8. **Monounsaturated Fatty Acids:**

9. **Polyunsaturated Fatty Acids:**

10. **Monounsaturated Fats:**

11. **Chylomicrons:**

12. **Very Low Density Lipoproteins (VLDL):**

13. **Essential Fatty Acids:**

14. **Essential Amino Acids:**

## Match the Following Terms

1. _____Monosaccharides

2. _____Disaccharides

3. _____Polysaccharides

4. _____Complex Carbohydrates

5. _____Glycogen

6. _____Starch

7. _____Fiber

8. _____Glucose

9. _____Fructose

10. _____Galactose

11. _____Lactose

12. _____Maltose

13. _____Sucrose

a) The main storage form of carbohydrate found primarily in the liver and muscles.

b) A simple sugar (monosaccharide) found in dairy products.

c) A simple sugar (monosaccharide) used as the primary fuel source by most cells in the body to generate energy.

d) The most simple form of carbohydrates comprised of one saccharide molecule.

e) A disaccharide found in many plants and used as a sweetener; commonly known as table sugar.

f) A complex carbohydrate found in seeds, fruits, and stems of plants and more notably in corn, rice, potatoes, and wheat.

g) A simple form of carbohydrate comprised of two monosaccharides.

h) Indigestible plant matter, consisting primarily of polysaccharides, that when consumed increase water absorption and intestinal peristalsis.

i) A white sugar formed during the digestion of starch.

j) A sweet sugar (monosaccharide) found primarily in fruits.

k) Sugar molecules that are strung together in long complex chains.

l) A disaccharide in dairy products that hydrolyzes to yield glucose and galactose.

m) A simple form of carbohydrate consisting of a number of monosaccharides.

## Fill in the Blanks with Appropriate Terms

1. _____ is a rating system for evaluating how different foods affect blood sugar levels.

2. The increment in energy expenditure above resting metabolic rate due to the cost of processing food for storage and use is known as the _____ .

3. The _____ mechanism refers to the body's preferential utilization of fats and carbohydrates instead of protein for energy.

4. Oils or fats called _____ contain one or two different types of compounds.

5. A _____ fat, most often of animal origin, is solid at room temperature and negatively affects blood levels of LDL cholesterol.

6. _____ is a high lipid complex containing protein that functions as a transporter of cholesterol in blood, which at high levels is associated with an increased risk of atherosclerosis and coronary heart disease (CHD).

7. An unsaturated fatty acid produced by the partial hydrogenation of vegetable oil is referred to as a

_____ .

8. _____ is an Omega-3 and _____ is an Omega-6 unsaturated fatty acid, both considered essential to the human diet.

9. A _____ is a food source that contains adequate amounts of the essential amino acids, while _____ are food sources that do not contain adequate amounts of every essential amino acid.

## Competency Exercises

1. Name the six classes of nutrients and whether they are energy or non-energy yielding.

1. _____
2. _____
3. _____
4. _____
5. _____
6. _____

2. Identify the different types of carbohydrates and provide an example of each.

**Type of Carbohydrate**                          **Example**

_____          _____

_____          _____

_____          _____

3. Identify three sources of fiber and the recommended daily intake requirement.

    1. _____

    2. _____

    3. _____


            Recommended Daily Intake Requirement: _____


4. Glucose synthesis in the liver is done via a process called _____.


5. Give the recommended percentage of carbohydrate in the diet for each activity status.

    Sedentary individual -                          _____ %

    Individual who exercises regularly -            _____ %

    Individual who does regular intense training -  _____ %


6. Fill in the following chart.

| Population | Carbohydrate Recommendation |
| --- | --- |
| Sedentary Individual | _____g/kg of body weight |
| Physically Active | _____g/kg of body weight |
| Moderate Exercise | _____g/kg of body weight |
| Vigorous Exercise | _____g/kg of body weight |


7. Identify five important functions of fat in the body.

    1. _____

    2. _____

    3. _____

    4. _____

    5. _____

8. Give the recommended intake for each lipid group.

| Lipid Classification | Recommended Intake |
|---|---|
| Dietary Fat | ≤ _____% total diet |
| Saturated Fat | ≤ _____% total diet |
| Monounsaturated Fat | _____% total diet |
| Polyunsaturated Fat | _____% total diet |
| Cholesterol | ≤ _____mg/day |
| Trans Fat | < _____% total diet |

9. There are _____ different kinds of amino acids, _____ are considered essential for adults and 9 for children.

10. Fill in the following chart.

| Population | Recommended Protein Intake |
|---|---|
| Sedentary Individual | _____ g/kg of body weight |
| Physically Active | _____ g/kg of body weight |
| Endurance Athlete | _____ g/kg of body weight |
| Bodybuilding & Strength Training | _____ g/kg of body weight |
| Children | Up to _____ g/kg of body weight |
| Pregnant Female | Add _____ g to total daily requirements<br>Add _____ g if nursing |

11. Approximately _____ % to _____ % of total calories in the diet should come from proteins.

12. Calculate your daily protein requirement in calories.

_____ x _____ g/kg of protein = _____ g/day

## Lesson Seven Quiz Questions

1. An individual's nutritional need is based on which of the following?

    A.  Relative genetic predisposition
    B.  Meeting specific requirements of energy expenditure
    C.  Dietary preferences
    D.  Variations in nutrient digestion, absorption, and assimilation.
    E.  All of the above

2. Which of the following represents the storage form of carbohydrate in humans?

    A.  Minerals
    B.  Starch
    C.  Glycogen
    D.  Vitamins

3. Fiber directly aids in all of the following except:

    A.  Gastrointestinal functioning
    B.  Mobilizing harmful chemicals
    C.  Protein synthesis
    D.  Slowing the absorption rate of carbohydrates

4. Long-term weight loss stimulated by short-term dieting is only effective approximately _____ % of the time.

    A.  <5
    B.  10
    C.  20
    D.  30

5. Diets high in _____ have been linked with increased coronary risk.

    A.  Cholesterol
    B.  Saturated fats
    C.  Trans fatty Acids
    D.  All of the above

6. Protein intakes above 2.0 g/kg of body weight may cause which of the following negative side effects?

    A.  Increased renal stress
    B.  Increased lipid storage
    C.  Dehydration
    D.  All of the above

*Answers  1 E, 2 C, 3 C, 4 A, 5 D, 6 D*

# Lesson Eight
# Nutrition: Non-Energy Yielding Nutrients

## Learning Objectives

- Define the role and function of fat and water soluble vitamins
- Discuss the possible negative effects associated with excessive vitamin consumption
- Identify the basic nutrient recommendations of the four categorical sets of reference values of the Dietary Reference Intakes (DRI's)
- Explain the general role and function of minerals in the body
- Explain the relationship between free radicals and antioxidants
- List antioxidant nutrients
- Describe the functions of calcium in the body
- Identify the recommended dietary intake of calcium for men, women, and children and the potential consequences of inadequate consumption
- Explain the role iron serves in oxygen transportation and the consequences of iron deficiency
- List the three components of the female triad
- Describe the role of electrolytes in the body
- Explain the relationship between water and minerals and the ability to regulate normal bodily function
- Explain the importance of fluid maintenance in the body
- Discuss conditions in which fluid is lost via metabolic demands, environmental temperature regulation, and exercise
- Identify the different signs and symptoms indicating dehydration
- Describe appropriate methods for maintaining hydration during exercise
- Describe the role of the United States Department of Agriculture (USDA) Food Guide Pyramid and the U.S. Dietary Guidelines in making healthy nutritional choices
- Assess food labels relative to serving size, nutrient value, and energy content

---

## Fill in the Blanks with Appropriate Terms

1. An amino acid called _____ is normally used by the body in cellular metabolism and to manufacture proteins. Elevated concentrations in the blood are thought to increase the risks for heart disease.

2. A(n) _____ is a type of bone cell that removes bone tissue by removing the

   bone's mineralized matrix, while _____ are cells from which bone develops.

3. A condition often seen in female athletes known as the _____ presents with three main conditions: disordered eating, amenorrhea, and osteoporosis.

4. The establishment of a proper electrical gradient across cell membranes called the

   _____ helps to regulate fluid balance in the tissues thus maintaining homeostasis.

5. _____ is a condition in which the body is in constant deprivation of fluids necessary for the maintenance of homeostasis and can result in debilitating conditions such as gastritis, heartburn, arthritis, kidney stones, and accelerated aging.

6.  A diagram used in nutrition education referred to as the _____ shows the suggested quantity of food from each food group that an individual should consume each day.

7.  The _____ is a label on consumer products that identifies servings per container, amount of food by weight or volume that constitutes a single serving, and relevant nutritional information.

8.  The _____ indicates the amount of a nutrient that is provided by a single serving of a food item.

## Match the Following Terms

1.  _____ Water-soluble Vitamins

2.  _____ Fat-soluble Vitamins

3.  _____ Coenzymes

4.  _____ Antioxidants

5.  _____ Free Radicals

6.  _____ Minerals

7.  _____ Calcium

8.  _____ Iron

9.  _____ Electrolytes

10. _____ Aldosterone

a)  Any of a group of inorganic elements that are essential to humans and animals for normal body function.

b)  Salts and minerals that produce electrically charged particles (ions) in the body fluids and are an important component in maintaining proper hydration status.

c)  An unstable molecule that causes oxidative damage by stealing electrons from surrounding molecules, thereby disrupting activity in the body's cells.

d)  Consist of the vitamins A, D, E, and K.

e)  A steroid hormone secreted by the adrenal cortex that regulates the salt and water balance in the body.

f)  Consists of the B-vitamins and vitamin C and are stored in the body for a brief period of time before being excreted.

g)  A key mineral in the formation of oxygen binding material including hemoglobin and myoglobin.

h)  A mineral essential in building and maintaining bone, as well as blood clotting and muscle contraction.

i)  A non-protein organic substance that usually contains a vitamin or mineral and combines with a specific protein, the apoenzyme, to form an active enzyme system.

j)  A chemical compound or substance thought to protect the body's cells from the damaging effects of oxidation that occurs as a result of free radical activity.

## Define the Following Terms

1.  **Dietary Reference Intakes (DRI):**

2.  **Estimated Average Requirements (EAR):**

3.  **Recommended Daily Allowance (RDA):**

4.  **Adequate Intakes (AI):**

5.  **Tolerable Upper Intake Levels (UL):**

6.  **Dehydration:**

7.  **Hypovolemia:**

8. **Osmolarity**:

9. **Food Description**:

10. **Nutrient Content**:

## Competency Exercises

1. What are the two classifications of vitamins?

    1. _____

    2. _____

2. List three vitamins that can help protect the body against free radical activity.

    1. _____

    2. _____

    3. _____

3. List four functions of minerals in the body.

    1. _____

    2. _____

    3. _____

    4. _____

4. What is the key mineral in the formation of oxygen binding material. _____

5. Water makes up about _____ % of muscle weight and _____ % of fat weight.

    1. 65, 55
    2. 75, 50
    3. 50, 75
    4. 80, 40

6. List five characteristics, signs, or symptoms of the female triad.

    1. _____

    2. _____

    3. _____

    4. _____

    5. _____


7. List four mechanisms by which fluid is lost through the body.

    1. _____

    2. _____

    3. _____

    4. _____


8. Briefly explain how the intensity of exercise can be affected by heat and humidity.

_____

_____

_____


9. List 8 early warning signs of dehydration.

    1. _____

    2. _____

    3. _____

    4. _____

    5. _____

    6. _____

    7. _____

    8. _____

10. The initiation of thirst occurs at a level of approximately _____ % loss of body weight from water.

    1.  0.1-0.6
    2.  0.8-2.0
    3.  2.1-3.2
    4.  3.4-4.6

11. Pre-exercise fluid consumption (30-60 min pre exercise) should be approximately _____ ml of water.

    1.  100-300
    2.  200-400
    3.  400-600
    4.  600-800

12. Provide three possible meanings for the term *light* listed on a food label.

    1.  _____

    2.  _____

    3.  _____

**Lesson Eight Quiz Questions**

1. Which of the following reacts with free radicals to prevent cellular damage?

    A. Proteins
    B. Carbohydrates
    C. Antioxidants
    D. Fatty acids

2. What mineral functions to support the integrity of bone and facilitates muscle contractions?

    A. Iron
    B. Selenium
    C. Calcium
    D. Potassium

3. In general, a sedentary person in normal environmental conditions should consume approximately _____ L of water each day.

    A. 1.0-1.5
    B. 2.0-2.5
    C. 3.0-3.5
    D. 4.0-4.5

4. Which of the following is a water-soluble antioxidant?

    A. Vitamin D
    B. Vitamin E
    C. Selenium
    D. Vitamin C

5. What is the most common mineral deficiency worldwide?

    A. Iron
    B. Sodium
    C. Potassium
    D. Calcium

*Answers 1 C, 2 C, 3 B, 4 D, 5 A*

# Lesson Nine
# Nutritional Supplementation

## Learning Objectives

- Describe the appropriate means for maximizing glycogen storage before competition
- Explain the difference, in terms, between supplements and ergogenic aids
- Identify the role the FDA plays in the regulation of supplements
- Explain the possible effects of creatine supplementation on performance
- Define the role of branched chain amino acids
- Describe the function and regulation of glutamine in the body
- Explain the role of L-arginine in the body
- Describe the primary function of nitric oxide in the body
- Explain the perceived benefit of using HMB and what conclusive evidence there might be to back the claims
- Identify concerns related to ingesting prohormones
- Discuss the allure some athletes have in taking androgenic-anabolic steroids and the potential adverse side effects associated with their use
- Describe the purported effects of weight loss supplements on the body's energy level, metabolism, appetite, and fat regulation
- Discuss the potential positive effects associated with caffeine intake and consequences of over consumption
- Identify possible negative side effects of ephedra and bitter orange
- Describe the mechanism for weight loss of Sibutramine and Orlistat

## Fill in the Blanks with Appropriate Terms

1. _____ are a group of anti-inflammatory, steroid-like compounds such as hydrocortisone that are produced by the adrenal cortex.

2. An enlargement of the cardiac muscle is known as _____.

3. Diseases or disorders of the heart muscle of unknown cause are called _____.

4. _____ are intraglandular precursors of hormones.

5. Any of various connective tissue cells found in the adipose tissue are called

   _____, which specialize in the storage of fat.

6. A drug labeled _____ suppresses the appetite by altering the body's

   metabolism, while _____ is a drug that suppresses appetite by inhibiting the reuptake of the neurotransmitters norepinephrine and serotonin.

## Define the Following Terms

1. **Atrophy**:

2. **Vasodilator**:

3.  **Delayed Onset Muscle Soreness (DOMS):**

4.  **Jaundice:**

5.  **Bronchodilator:**

6.  **Orlistat:**

7.  **Dopamine:**

8.  **Norepinephrine:**

9.  **Serotonin:**

## Match the Following Terms

1.  _____Supplement

2.  _____Ergogenic aids

3.  _____Creatine monohydrate

4.  _____Glutamine

5.  _____Nitric oxide

6.  _____HMB

7.  _____Alanine

8.  _____L-arginine

9.  _____Androgenic Anabolic Steroids

10. _____Dehydroepiandrosterone (DHEA)

11. _____Caffeine

12. _____Guarana

13. _____Amphetamines

a)  A non-essential amino acid that is a constituent of many proteins.

b)  A class of natural and synthetic steroid hormones that promote cell growth and division, resulting in growth of several types of tissues, especially muscle and bone.

c)  A natural substance similar to caffeine.

d)  A nitrogenous organic acid that is found in the muscle tissue in the form of phosphocreatine and supplies energy for muscle contraction.

e)  Any one of a group of drugs that are powerful central nervous system stimulants.

f)  A substance added to the diet to make up for a deficiency.

g)  A compound involved in oxygen transport to the tissues, the transmission of nerve impulses, and other physiological activities, chiefly as a vasodilator.

h)  Any external influences which can positively affect physical performance or mental focus.

i)  An alkaloid often found in tea or coffee and used chiefly as a stimulant.

j)  A natural steroid hormone produced from cholesterol by the adrenal glands.

k)  A non-essential amino acid that occurs widely in proteins, blood, and other tissues.

l)  An amino acid obtained from the hydrolysis or digestion of protein.

m) A compound that minimizes the breakdown of proteins and damage to muscle cells.

## Competency Exercises

1. True or False? Protein is the only nutrient that should be consumed post-exercise.

2. True or False? Ingesting additional vitamins and minerals above the UL may increase the risk of toxicity poisoning in the tissues.

3. Provide three plausible reasons why individuals should be cautious when using supplements.

     1. _____

     2. _____

     3. _____

4. List four common supplements marketed as ergogenic aids.

     1. _____

     2. _____

     3. _____

     4. _____

5. Name three functions creatine has within the body.

     1. _____

     2. _____

     3. _____

6. Identify three negative effects of increased branched chain amino acid consumption.

     1. _____

     2. _____

     3. _____

7. List four potential positive effects of supplementing glutamine.

     1. _____

     2. _____

     3. _____

     4. _____

8. List four functions of L-arginine in the body.

    1. _____

    2. _____

    3. _____

    4. _____

9. Nitric oxide assists in the metabolic regulation of what three things?

    1. _____

    2. _____

    3. _____

10. List eight adverse side effects of steroid abuse.

    1. _____

    2. _____

    3. _____

    4. _____

    5. _____

    6. _____

    7. _____

    8. _____

11. True or False? Steroid abuse only has physiological side effects.

12. True or False? As a whole, weight loss supplements are very effective for long-term results.

13. Weight loss supplements are classified into five general categories that produce which five desired effects on the body?

    1. _____

    2. _____

    3. _____

    4. _____

    5. _____

14. Name two natural weight loss supplements widely used for weight reduction and performance enhancement.

    1. _____

    2. _____


15. List the two most common weight loss drugs.

    1. _____

    2. _____

## Lesson Nine Quiz Questions

1. What is the key component in the formation and repair of muscle fibers?

    A. Fiber
    B. Protein
    C. Carbohydrates
    D. Nitric Oxide

2. Which of the following is a non-essential amino acid alleged to be a growth hormone stimulator?

    A. L-arginine
    B. Glutamine
    C. Valine
    D. Leucine

3. Which of the following negative effects can result from steroid abuse?

    A. Elevated blood pressure
    B. Myocardial hypertrophy
    C. Depression of serum high-density lipoproteins
    D. All of the above

4. _____ is a widely-used, naturally occurring weight loss supplement.

    A. Orlistat
    B. Caffeine
    C. Aspirin
    D. Mazindol

5. It is estimated that a harmful response to ephedra use occurs in about 1 per _____ people.

    A. 10
    B. 100
    C. 1000
    D. 10,000

*Answers  1 B, 2 A, 3 D, 4 B, 5 C*

## Lesson Ten
## Body Composition

### Learning Objectives

- Define body composition and explain how values are used to quantify fat mass and fat-free mass on the body
- Identify essential body fat values for men and women and explain the role essential fat levels play in the body
- Discuss the relationship between body composition and health
- Describe the health implications of different types of body fat distribution patterns
- Explain the role of hormones and androgenic receptors in human adiposity
- Identify limitations of height weight tables in determining ideal weight
- Calculate Body Mass Index and explain its role in predicting disease risk
- Implement methods used for circumference measurements and explain how they are used to predict obesity-related risk for disease
- Identify effective methods for body composition assessment and discuss benefits and limitations associated with each
- Perform skinfold analysis and girth measurements to determine body composition
- Identify healthy body composition values and those that define obesity
- Calculate target body weight using measured body fat percentage

### Match the Following Terms

1. _____ Body Mass Index (BMI)

2. _____ Essential Body Fat

3. _____ Subcutaneous Fat

4. _____ Visceral Fat

5. _____ Android Obesity

6. _____ Gynoid Obesity

7. _____ Body Composition

8. _____ Circumference Measurements

9. _____ Skinfold Measurements

10. _____ Cellulite

a) Used to describe the percentages of fat and lean mass in human bodies; the relationship of fat mass to fat free mass.

b) Fat stored in and around the organs.

c) A non-invasive estimation of body composition employed by measuring the girth of select locations to predict body fat; ideal for obese populations.

d) A fatty deposit causing a dimpled or uneven surface of the skin.

e) A measure which takes into account a person's weight and height. The main purpose is to predict health consequences.

f) The most widely used body composition testing method to assess body fat percentage; ideal for fit populations.

g) Fat required for normal physiological functioning.

h) Male pattern or abdominal fat storage associated with an "apple-shaped" physique.

i) Fat just below the skin, measured with skinfold assessment.

j) Female pattern or gluteal fat storage associated with a "pear-shaped" physique.

## Fill in the Blanks with Appropriate Terms

1.  A condition called _____ is present when there are excessive levels of circulating insulin in the blood.

2.  _____ are cell receptors which increase the release of free fatty acids from adipose storage in response to catecholamines.

3.  _____ are cell receptors which reduce the lipolytic response to catecholamines.

4.  A formula used to assist in setting short- and long-term weight loss goals is the

    _____ .

## Define the Following Terms

1.  **Height Weight Tables (HWT):**

2.  **Waist-to-Hip ratio (WHR):**

3.  **Dual X-ray Absorptiometry (DXA):**

4.  **Bioelectrical Impedance Analysis (BIA):**

5.  **Near-infrared (NIR) Light Interactance:**

## Competency Exercises

1. According to the Department of Health and Human Services, the incidence of what five heart-related diseases increases with a BMI > 25.

    1. _____

    2. _____

    3. _____

    4. _____

    5. _____

2. Essential body fat levels for males are _____ .

    1.  1 – 2 %
    2.  3 – 5 %
    3.  6 – 8 %
    4.  9 – 12 %

3. Essential body fat levels for females are _____ .

    1.  5 – 8 %
    2.  9 – 10 %
    3.  11 – 14 %
    4.  15 – 18 %

4. What four variables account for the storage of adipose tissue in the body?

    1. _____

    2. _____

    3. _____

    4. _____

5. Upper body fat storage is associated with what three common health risks?

    1. _____

    2. _____

    3. _____

6. Give a brief explanation of why there is a difference in fat distribution between sexes.

_____

_____

_____

_____

7. Which fat pattern, male or female is more easily altered or reduced?

_____Why? _____

8. Provide the original basis for using height-weight tables and provide tow possible problems with the table published by the USDA.

    1. _____

    2. _____

9. List four considerations when using the Metropolitan Life height weight tables.

    1. _____

    2. _____

    3. _____

    4. _____

10. Fill in the following equation for Body Mass Index.

BMI = _____ ÷ _____

11. During the accurate measurement of hip to waist ratio, identify where each measurement should be taken for the specific location.

Hip measurement- _____

Waist Measurement- _____

12. Waist-to-Hip ratios present the greatest risk when values are above _____ in men and _____ in women.

1.  0.6;0.7
2.  0.7;0.6
3.  0.8;0.9
4.  0.9;0.8

13. Briefly explain why body composition assessments are important to personal trainers.

_____

_____

_____

14. Give three common clinical body composition tests.

1. _____

2. _____

3. _____

15. Give four common body composition field tests.

1. _____

2. _____

3. _____

4. _____

16. Give three reasons why clinical assessments are not commonly used in personal training settings.

1. _____

2. _____

3. _____

17. True of False? Skinfold assessments should be performed on individuals who are not visibly obese.

18. Match the body composition exam with the brief description given.

    1. _____Circumference measurements          a) assessment based on water conductivity

    2. _____Skinfold measurements                b) measures select locations to predict body fat

    3. _____Bioelectrical impedance               c) assesses tissue makeup using light emissions

    4. _____Near-infrared light interactance       d) technicians pinch select sites to assess fat

19. Give four factors where error may occur when using Bioelectrical Impedance analysis.

    1. _____

    2. _____

    3. _____

    4. _____

20. Fill in the following target body weight formula.

Fat mass = current body weight X (% body fat ÷ 100 )

Fat-free mass (FFM) = current body weight – fat mass

Target body weight = $\dfrac{FFM}{1 - \dfrac{\{Desired\ \%\ BF\}}{100}}$

         Fat mass = _____ X (% _____ ÷ _____ )

         Fat-free mass (FFM) = _____ – _____

         Target body weight =

$$\dfrac{(\quad\quad)}{1 - \{\dfrac{\quad\quad\%\quad\quad}{100}\}}$$

## Lesson Ten Quiz Questions

1. Subcutaneous fat represents approximately _____% of total fat stored in the body.

    A. 20-40 %
    B. 30-50 %
    C. 40-60 %
    D. 50-70 %

2. A waist circumference above _____ inches for males is associated with cardiovascular and metabolic disease.

    A. 30
    B. 40
    C. 50
    D. 60

3. Which body composition test would be most appropriate for a personal trainer?

    A. Skinfold Assessment
    B. Hydrostatic weighing
    C. Air displacement plethsmography
    D. Dual x-ray absorptiometry

4. Skinfold estimation error is most commonly attributed to testing error by the technician due to:

    A. Inexperience
    B. Variations in tissue consistency
    C. Too much fat mass at the site
    D. Incorrect site identification
    E. All of the above

5. All of the following are bioelectrical impedance testing guidelines except:

    A. No eating or drinking within 4 hours of the test
    B. Don't void the bowel or bladder immediately before assessment
    C. No alcohol consumption for more than 24 hours
    D. Avoid testing during female menstruation

*Answers  1 D, 2 B, 3 A, 4 E, 5 B*

# Lesson Eleven
# Weight Management

## Learning Objectives

- Identify the prevalence of overweight and obesity in the United States
- Recognize the factors that positively and negatively affect successful weight management
- Identify the role energy balance plays in weight management
- Explain why significant caloric restriction can negatively affect lean mass
- Demonstrate competency in the implementation of dietary assessment protocols and identify common errors in data collection
- Calculate resting metabolic rate and explain its role in determining daily caloric need
- Recognize possible errors in determining daily caloric need and how each may affect energy balance
- Identify effective dietary and physical activity strategies to meet weight management goals
- Explain why spot reduction of adipose tissue is unattainable
- Explain how social behaviors may positively or negatively affect weight management attempts
- Provide sound methods in weight gain
- Identify problems with fad diets and why they rarely end in successful long-term weight loss
- Identify types of eating disorders and common characteristics of each

---

## Match the Following Terms

1. _____Hypothalamus

2. _____Very low calorie diet (VLCD)

3. _____Resting Metabolic Rate (RMR)

4. _____Cunningham Lean Mass Equation

5. _____Revised Harris-Benedict Equations

6. _____Excess post-exercise oxygen consumption (EPOC)

7. _____Total energy expenditure (TEE)

8. _____Anorexia Nervosa

9. _____Bulimia Nervosa

10. _____Binge-eating disorder

a)  A measurably increased rate of oxygen intake following strenuous activity.

b)  The rate at which the body expends energy to support vital functions including heart contractions, digestion, and various cellular contractions at rest.

c)  A psychiatric and medical condition which involves an individual engaging in episodes of binge eating followed by various efforts to "purge" or expel the binged food.

d)  Regulates body temperature, certain metabolic processes, and other autonomic activities.

e)  A psycho-physiological disorder, characterized by fear of becoming obese, a distorted self image, a persistent aversion to food, and severe weight loss.

f)  An equation used to predict resting metabolic rate (RMR) which may be more appropriate when lean mass cannot be accurately determined.

g)  A diet of 800 kilocalories a day or less.

h)  The overall amount of energy used throughout the day for activity and vital body functions; a combination of RMR plus voluntary metabolism and thermic effect of food.

i)  A recurrent eating disorder characterized by the uncontrolled, excessive intake of any available food which often occurs following stressful events.

j)  An equation used to predict resting metabolic rate (RMR) when an individual's body composition has been accurately identified.

## Competency Exercises

1.  Very low calorie diets (VLCD) usually contain between _____ - _____ calories.

    1.   400-800
    2.   800-1200
    3.   1200-1600
    4.   1400-1800

2. Give four problems or errors commonly encountered when logging food intake.

    1.  _____

    2.  _____

    3.  _____

    4.  _____

3. For each of the following components of caloric expenditure, provide the approximate percentage that reflects the relative contribution from each.

    Resting metabolic rate-   _____%

    Physical activity-      _____%

    Thermic effect of food-   _____%

4. Identify six factors that contribute to metabolic rate.

    1.  _____

    2.  _____

    3.  _____

    4.  _____

    5.  _____

    6.  _____

5. What RMR estimation equation would be most accurate for a young, lean individual?

    _____

6. List three controllable factors or variables that can lead to either weight loss or gain.

1. _____

2. _____

3. _____

7. True or False? Individuals who are sedentary except for the 30 - 40 minutes of exercise they perform three days a week may actually have a greater risk for weight gain than a person who does not engage in any structured exercise, but is physically active throughout the week.

8. Provide three examples of exercise alternatives that could be incorporated into everyday life to increase daily physical activity.

1. _____

2. _____

3. _____

9. True or False? Exercise aimed at weight loss should only include aerobic activities.

10. Name seven strategies for weight loss.

1. _____

2. _____

3. _____

4. _____

5. _____

6. _____

7. _____

11. Explain how stress can affect weight management outcomes.

_____

_____

_____

_____

12. True or False? Diagnosed eating disorders are classified as psychological disorders.

13. List five common characteristics of eating disorders.

    1. _____

    2. _____

    3. _____

    4. _____

    5. _____


14. Identify the three most common eating disorders and provide a brief description of each.

_____        _____

                              _____

_____        _____

                              _____

_____        _____

                              _____

## Lesson Eleven Quiz Questions

1. Exercise aimed at weight loss should focus on _____.

    A.  High intensity aerobic training
    B.  Resistance training
    C.  Caloric expenditure
    D.  Exercise in the fat-burning zone

2. The use of equations to predict resting metabolic rate (RMR) are based on which of the following principles?

    A.  RMR is proportionate to body size
    B.  RMR decreases with age
    C.  Muscle is more metabolically active than fat
    D.  All of the above

3. It is estimated that the addition of one pound of lean mass represents approximately _____ calories expended during rest per day.

    A.  3-6
    B.  7-10
    C.  11-15
    D.  16-19

4. The caloric density of alcohol is ____ kcals per gram.

    A.  4
    B.  5
    C.  6
    D.  7

5. Dietary intake of calories should not drop below _____ without medical supervision.

    A.  800
    B.  1200
    C.  1500
    D.  2000

*Answers  1 C, 2 D, 3 C, 4 D, 5 B*

# Lesson Twelve
# Physical Fitness & Health

## Learning Objectives

- Explain the difference between health and wellness
- Identify factors that positively and negatively affect one's health
- Define the health-related components of fitness and the respective role of each in disease prevention and optimal health attainment
- Define the performance-related components of fitness and the respective role of each in human performance and function
- Explain the difference between health and physical fitness
- Identify factors that affect baseline measures of physical fitness
- Explain the relationship between physical activity and health-related quality of life
- Identify the risks associated with engaging in physical activity and the role pre-exercise screening plays in reducing risk of an adverse event
- Identify the role physical activity plays; the type of activity that promotes improvement; and the dose-response relationship for each of the following diseases or conditions: Cardiovascular Disease, Coronary Artery Disease, Atherosclerosis, Hypertension, Obesity, Stroke, Diabetes, Osteoarthritis, Osteoporosis, Cancer, Mental Health

## Match the Following Terms

1. _____ Hyperlipidemia

2. _____ Cardiorespiratory fitness (CRF)

3. _____ Tendonitis

4. _____ Plantar fasciitis

5. _____ Epicondylitis

6. _____ Hyperthermia

7. _____ Hypothermia

8. _____ Hypoglycemia

9. _____ Rhabdomyolysis

10. _____ Cardiovascular disease (CVD)

11. _____ Coronary heart disease (CHD)

12. _____ Arrhythmias

13. _____ Thrombosis

a) An abnormally low level of glucose in the blood.

b) An abnormal heart rhythm.

c) A general diagnostic category consisting of several separate diseases of the heart and circulatory system.

d) An excess of fats or lipids circulating in the blood.

e) Formation of a blood clot in the heart or blood vessel.

f) Refers to the ability of the circulatory and respiratory systems to supply oxygen to working muscles during sustained activity.

g) Inflammation of a tendon.

h) An inflammatory condition caused by excessive wear to the plantar fascia (bottom of the foot).

i) Progressive reduction of blood supply to the heart due to narrowing or blocking of the coronary artery.

j) Inflammation of the muscles and soft tissues around an epicondyle.

k) An acute, potentially fatal disease that destroys skeletal muscle and is often accompanied by the excretion of myoglobin in the urine.

l) Unusually high body temperature.

m) Abnormally low body temperature.

## Fill in the Blanks with Appropriate Terms

1. The harmonious adjustment or interaction of parts controlled by the nervous system is commonly referred to as

   _____.

2. _____ refers to the body's ability to change direction.

3. The clean, jerk, and snatch exercises are known as _____.

4. _____ are exercises that use explosive movements to develop muscular power.

5. The science of biological inheritance is called _____. It contributes to the measurable components of physical fitness during a person's lifespan and also helps to determine the potential capabilities of the body.

6. Usually referred to as type I diabetes, _____, is an autoimmune disorder in which the body's own immune system attacks the pancreas.

7. Usually referred to as type II diabetes, _____, is a metabolic disorder characterized by insulin resistance, an insulin deficiency, and hyperglycemia, often related to poor diet and limited physical activity.

8. A form of arthritis called _____ occurs mainly in older individuals and is characterized by chronic degradation of the cartilage in the joints.

## Define the Following Terms

1. **Diuretics:**

2. **Beta-Blockers:**

3. **Angiostensin Converting Enzyme (ACE) Inhibitors:**

4. **Calcium Channel Blockers:**

5. **Alpha-Blockers:**

6. **Nervous System Inhibitors:**

7. **Vasodilators:**

## Competency Exercises

1. Identify six health components related to physical fitness.

    1. _____

    2. _____

    3. _____

    4. _____

    5. _____

    6. _____

3. True or False? Body composition is the actual amount of fat a person maintains on his or her body.

2. Identify five performance components related to physical fitness.

    1. _____

    2. _____

    3. _____

    4. _____

    5. _____

4. List 4 factors that contribute to an individual's overall physical fitness.

    1. _____

    2. _____

    3. _____

    4. _____

5. List a frequent injury common for each of the following activities.

    Jogging        _____

    Bicycling      _____

    Swimming     _____

    Aerobic dance  _____

    Tennis         _____

6. It is estimated that the number of deaths associated with a sedentary lifestyle is approximately _____ annually.

    A. 100,000
    B. 200,000
    C. 300,000
    D. 400,000

7. Aerobic exercise has a positive effect on several factors that influence risk for cardiovascular disease including reductions in:

    1. _____

    2. _____

    3. _____

    4. _____

    5. _____

8. Smokers are at _____ % greater risk for heart disease than non-smokers.

    A. 40
    B. 50
    C. 60
    D. 70

9. Endurance trained athletes generally have _____ more circulating HDL cholesterol than same aged sedentary, but healthy individuals.

    A. 10 – 20 %
    B. 20 – 30 %
    C. 30 – 40 %
    D. 40 – 50 %

10. True or False? Moderate intensity and high intensity activity have been shown to yield the same benefits in HDL production as long as adequate energy expenditure is met.

11. Cardiac events related to coronary heart disease are often triggered by which two separate complications?

    1. _____

    2. _____

12. Name five health problems and complications related to hypertension.

    1. _____

    2. _____

    3. _____

    4. _____

    5. _____

13. Exercise guidelines for reducing hypertension.

    _____

14. Give the ranges for systolic and diastolic measures in each specified category.

| | Systolic | Diastolic |
|---|---|---|
| Optimal Blood Pressure | $\leq$ _____ | $\leq$ _____ |
| Normal Blood Pressure | < _____ | < _____ |
| Pre-hypertension | _____ - _____ | _____ - _____ |
| Hypertension | $\geq$ _____ | $\geq$ _____ |
| BP Medical Referral | $\geq$ _____ | $\geq$ _____ |

15. Obesity is a risk factor associated with what diseases (name six)?

    1. _____

    2. _____

    3. _____

    4. _____

    5. _____

    6. _____

16. What component must accompany calorie control to yield the best results for weight loss?

    _____

17. Physical activity using non-impact resistance and aerobic modalities performed at moderate levels has been shown in osteoarthritis patients to:

1. _____

2. _____

3. _____

18. What three positive self-reported effects might moderate intensity activity have on osteoarthritic clients?

1. _____

2. _____

3. _____

19. Name three areas of the body that experience the greatest risk of injury due to osteoporosis.

1. _____

2. _____

3. _____

20. Which gender is at the greatest risk of developing osteoporosis? Give three explanations why.

_____ ; due to:

1. _____

2. _____

3. _____

21. True or False? Research has shown that physical activity has a pronounced effect on symptoms of depression, clinical depression, and anxiety.

## Lesson Twelve Quiz Questions

1. The body's ability to produce and sustain force output is known as _____.

   A. Cardiorespiratory Fitness
   B. Muscular Fitness
   C. Cardiopulmonary Fitness
   D. None of the above

2. The ability of the body to rapidly change direction is known as _____.

   A. Speed
   B. Quickness
   C. Agility
   D. Coordination

3. Physical activity is associated with a reduction in risk of which of the following diseases?

   A. Colon Cancer
   B. Hypertension
   C. Non-insulin dependent diabetes mellitus
   D. Coronary heart disease
   E. All of the above

4. Which of the following drugs acts on the kidneys to prevent the re-absorption of water?

   A. Calcium Channel Blockers
   B. Vasodilators
   C. Diuretics
   D. Beta-blockers

5. Currently about 1 of every ____ persons in the United States is classifiably hypertensive.

   A. 3
   B. 5
   C. 7
   D. 9

6. Which of the following is the key risk factor for developing osteoarthritis?

   A. Weight
   B. Activity Level
   C. Race
   D. Age

*Answers 1 B, 2 C, 3 E, 4 C, 5 A, 6 D*

# Lesson Thirteen
# Pre-Exercise Screening & Test Considerations

## Learning Objectives

- Explain the role of pre-exercise screening in determining physical activity participation
- Identify the proper procedure used to clear a participant for exercise
- Explain the components of the Informed Consent and how to properly implement the document
- Discuss the value of the Health Status Questionnaire and Behavior Questionnaire in assessing health status
- List the common components of the Resting Battery of Physical Tests used for exercise screening
- Perform resting measurements of heart rate and blood pressure and identify values that require medical referral for activity participation clearance
- Identify body composition and blood lipid measurements that are indicative of disease and those that require medical referral for activity participation clearance
- Recognize common signs and symptoms of disease which may prevent safe participation in physical activity
- List the purposes for exercise testing
- Identify exercise test selection criteria used to determine the fitness test employed
- Explain how to increase exercise test validity and reliability
- List methods or strategies that increase the safety of exercise testing
- Discuss the importance of proper test interpretation and its role in client motivation
- Explain how a Needs Analysis is constructed and how it is used in program development
- Explain the difference between short-term and long-term goals and how attainable goals are determined

## Define the Following Terms

1. **Informed Consent**:

2. **PAR-Q**:

3. **Health Risk Appraisal**:

4. **Medical History Questionnaire**:

5. **Health Status Questionnaire**:

6. **Emergency Medical Service (EMS)**:

## Match the Following Terms

1. _____Obesity

2. _____Heart Palpitations

3. _____Edema

4. _____Hypertension

5. _____Dyslipidemia

6. _____Coronary Artery Disease

7. _____Metabolic Disease

8. _____Asthma

9. _____Stroke

10. _____Hypotension

11. _____Dyspnea

12. _____Hemoptysis

13. _____Amenorrhea

14. _____Insomnia

a) A chronic respiratory disease, often arising from allergies and characterized by sudden recurring attacks of difficult breathing, chest constriction, and coughing.

b) A menstrual irregularity seen especially in women who are involved in regular high intensity exercise.

c) An abnormality of the amounts of lipids in the blood.

d) An unhealthy accumulation of body fat, usually 20% or more over an individual's ideal body weight.

e) Chronic inability to fall asleep or remain asleep for an adequate length of time.

f) An excessive accumulation of fluid in tissue spaces or a body cavity.

g) The sudden death of brain cells in a localized area due to inadequate blood flow.

h) A narrowing or blockage of the arteries and vessels that provide oxygen and nutrients to the heart.

i) Difficulty in breathing, often associated with lung or heart disease and resulting in shortness of breath.

j) A sensation in which a person is aware of an irregular, hard, or rapid heartbeat.

k) Any disorder that involves an alteration in the normal metabolism of carbohydrates, lipids, proteins, water, and nucleic acids; evidenced by various syndromes and diseases such as hypertension, hyperlipidemia, obesity, and diabetes.

l) Arterial disease in which high blood pressure is the primary symptom.

m) The coughing up of blood or bloody sputum from the lungs or airway.

n) Abnormally low blood pressure.

## Competency Exercises

1. List three documents that can be used by personal trainers for preliminary screening of clients prior to engaging in activity.

    1. _____

    2. _____

    3. _____

2. True or False? By law, clients who are exposed to, or may be subject to possible physical or psychological injury must give informed consent prior to participation in the described activities.

3. List five general categories of questions that should be included in a comprehensive questionnaire.

1. _____

2. _____

3. _____

4. _____

5. _____


4. List eight risk factors that trainers should pay particular attention to in the health screening evaluations.

1. _____

2. _____

3. _____

4. _____

5. _____

6. _____

7. _____

8. _____


5. When reviewing a client's HSQ, trainers should pay attention to what key risk factors.

1. _____

2. _____

3. _____

4. _____

5. _____

6. _____

7. _____

8. _____

6.  List seven assessments that should be completed during the resting battery of the physical assessment.

1. _____

2. _____

3. _____

4. _____

5. _____

6. _____

7. _____


7.  List four (detrimental) consequences for the body as a result of high blood pressure.

1. _____

2. _____

3. _____

4. _____


8. The diagnostic criteria for Stage 1 Hypertension is a diastolic value of _____ mmHg and/or a systolic value of _____ mmHg.

A.  70;130
B.  80;130
C.  80;140
D.  90;140

9. Men with greater than _____% body fat and women with greater than _____% body fat are considered morbidly obese and require a physician's referral before exercise testing can be performed.

A.  20, 30
B.  30, 40
C.  40, 50
D.  None of the above

10. Give five signs or symptoms for each of the following diseases.

Cardiovascular:

1. _____

2. _____

3. _____

4. _____

5. _____

Pulmonary:

1. _____

2. _____

3. _____

4. _____

5. _____

Metabolic:

1. _____

2. _____

3. _____

4. _____

5. _____

11. Explain the difference between disease risk classifications.

_____

_____

_____

12. List six variables a trainer should monitor to increase the validity of the exercise testing.

    1. _____

    2. _____

    3. _____

    4. _____

    5. _____

    6. _____

13. List six variables a trainer should monitor to increase the reliability of the exercise testing.

    1. _____

    2. _____

    3. _____

    4. _____

    5. _____

    6. _____

14. True or False? When testing a client, tests that produce fatigue should be placed at the beginning of the testing sequence.

15. Number in successive order the logical progression for tests administered to a client which produce fatigue (i.e. 1$^{st}$, 2$^{nd}$ ...).

    _____ Muscle endurance tests

    _____ Anaerobic capacity tests

    _____ Resting test or test of minimal fatigue

    _____ Aerobic tests

    _____ Strength and power tests

## Lesson Thirteen Quiz Questions

1. An informed consent should contain information that presents:

 A. Risks
 B. Benefits
 C. Rationale
 D. Expectations of the program components
 E. All of the above

2. Which of the following would **not** cause an elevation of resting heart rate values?

 A. Low stroke volumes
 B. Poor oxygen extraction capabilities
 C. High hemoglobin levels
 D. Unregulated stress hormones

3. Ideally, measures of resting blood pressure are recommended to be at, or below, _____.

 A. 105/70 mg/dl
 B. 115/75 mg/dl
 C. 125/85 mg/dl
 D. 135/80 mg/dl

4. Medical clearance is recommended for clients who present with all the following values except:

 A. LDL <135 mg/dl
 B. HDL < 40 mg/dl
 C. Total Cholesterol $\geq$ 240
 D. Cholesterol ratio $\geq$ 5

5. Which of the following is a sign or symptom of cardiovascular disease?

 A. Leg pain upon exertion
 B. Dyspnea
 C. Chest or left arm pain
 D. High resting heart rate
 E. All of the above

6. Which of the following is a sign or symptom of metabolic disease?

 A. High or low blood glucose
 B. Central adiposity
 C. Obesity
 D. All of the above

7. Which of the following data is necessary for identifying the most appropriate exercise tests for a client?

 A. Experience
 B. Capabilities
 C. Training Status
 D. Age and Gender
 E. All of the above

*Answers 1 E, 2 C, 3 B, 4 A, 5 E, 6 D, 7 E*

# Lesson Fourteen
# Assessment of Physical Fitness

## Learning Objectives

- Explain the difference between maximal and submaximal testing for cardiorespiratory fitness
- Identify goals for muscle strength ratios at each major joint of the body
- Discuss problems with one repetition maximum testing for strength
- Explain the role strength plays in muscular endurance testing
- Explain the difference between anaerobic power and anaerobic capacity
- Discuss problems with using sit-and-reach as an assessment for flexibility and explain why multiple joint assessment is necessary for flexibility testing
- Identify methods which increase the accuracy and value of body composition measures
- Implement and explain the role of the fitness test preparation checklist
- Discuss how individual factors affect exercise test selection
- Identify and implement common field tests for cardiorespiratory fitness, muscular strength, muscular endurance, muscular power, body composition, and flexibility

## Match the Following Terms

1. _____ $VO_2$max

2. _____ Muscular strength

3. _____ Muscular endurance

4. _____ Activities of daily living (ADL's)

5. _____ Anaerobic capacity

6. _____ Goniometer

7. _____ Hydrostatic weighing

8. _____ Air displacement plethysmography

a) An instrument used for measuring specific joint angles with full attainable range of motion.

b) Tested in an apparatus called the 'Bod Pod', this method measures an individual's body composition using air displacement to measure body volume.

c) The highest rate at which oxygen can be taken up and utilized by an individual during exercise.

d) A clinically analyzed method of determining an individual's body composition in which the individual is weighed in air and subsequently weighed in water of known density. The volume of the individual is equal to the loss of weight in the water divided by the density of water.

e) The ability of a person to exert a maximal quantifiable force against an object.

f) The ability of a person to sustain a continual muscular exertion over a given period of time.

g) The length of time that a muscle can perform an activity utilizing the anaerobic glycolytic pathway to generate ATP until fatigue.

h) Activities that require a baseline functional ability and are completed every day such as: sitting, standing, dressing, bathing, etc.

1. Provide four reasons why personal trainers rarely employ maximal testing protocols.

    1. _____

    2. _____

    3. _____

    4. _____

2. True or False? Testing for muscular fitness includes assessing a client's capacity for both muscular strength and endurance.

3. Identify one problem with strength and endurance testing.

    _____

4. True or False? Selecting higher repetition tests over 1RM or 3RM is recommended for the average healthy population.

5. Give three obvious risks associated with low repetition maximal tests with healthy populations.

    1. _____

    2. _____

    3. _____

6. If a client cannot perform at least _____ repetitions for a given endurance assessment, then a different test should be selected.

    1. 10
    2. 15
    3. 20
    4. 25

7. List four common errors observed during muscular fitness testing.

    1. _____

    2. _____

    3. _____

    4. _____

8. List the three most common muscular power tests for older adults.

    1. _____

    2. _____

    3. _____

9. The emphasis of anaerobic power and capacity is a measurement of biochemical assessments including:

    1. _____

    2. _____

    3. _____

10. True or False? As flexibility declines, subsequent physical activity status declines due to reduced movement capacity.

11. List three variables that may reduce the validity of the sit-and-reach assessment.

    1. _____

    2. _____

    3. _____

12. Give the four main factors related to the decision of using one body composition testing method above another.

    1. _____

    2. _____

    3. _____

    4. _____

13. Accuracy when doing body composition assessments is dependent upon what two factors with regard to the testing procedure?

    1. _____

    2. _____

14. In general, acceptable estimation of error should not be higher than _____ because it may change the client's fitness profile and affect appropriate decision making for the program.

    1.  2%
    2.  4%
    3.  6%
    4.  8%
    5.  None of the above

15. True or False? Girth measurements should be used on leaner individuals and skinfold assessments should be used on everyone else.

## Lesson Fourteen Quiz Questions

1. Which of the following tests could be administered to a healthy adult to determine their anaerobic capacity?

 A. A power step test
 B. A YMCA bench press test
 C. A push-up test
 D. A 1.5 mile steady-state test

2. $VO_2$max reflects the body's ability to:

 A. Intake oxygen
 B. Transport oxygen
 C. Utilize oxygen in the tissues
 D. A & B only
 E. All of the above

3. Due to the potential for musculoskeletal differences between muscle groups, it is recommended to use a minimum of _____ different strength and endurance tests to assess muscular fitness.

 A. 2
 B. 3
 C. 4
 D. 5

4. Which of the following tests would be most affected by client effort?

 A. 1.5 mile run test
 B. Paced abdominal curl-up test using a metronome
 C. YMCA bike test
 D. All of the above are equally affected

5. Which of the following components of fitness is most often underrepresented in many fitness evaluations, but actually requires numerous tests for accurate assessment?

 A. Strength
 B. Cardiovascular efficiency
 C. Flexibility
 D. Anaerobic Endurance

*Answers 1 A, 2 E, 3 B, 4 A, 5 C*

# Lesson Fifteen
# Exercise Programming Components

## Learning Objectives

- List and explain the principles of exercise program design
- Identify the role of an exercise warm-up and discuss the acute physiological responses to the activity
- Identify the different types of warm-ups and compare the role of each in an exercise prescription
- Explain the role of a cool down following exercise participation
- Discuss how the metabolic systems are used in program decision making for the exercise prescription
- Explain how proper exercise selection is determined in anaerobic and aerobic exercise programs
- Discuss the importance of skill acquisition when implementing the exercise selection
- List the general order of activities in a program utilizing concurrent aerobic and anaerobic training modalities
- Define the following and explain how each is determined in an exercise program: Training frequency, Training duration, Training intensity, Rest intervals, Training volume, Recovery periods
- Define the principles of exercise and the role of each in program development
- Discuss how individual factors determine the application of progressive overload in an exercise program
- List factors that affect the safety of the exercise program and discuss strategies to account for each

## Match the Following Terms

1. _____ Kinetics

2. _____ Calisthenics

3. _____ Proprioception

4. _____ Intensity

5. _____ Circuit Training

6. _____ Micro Trauma

7. _____ Frequency

8. _____ Duration

9. _____ Principle of Specificity

10. _____ Principle of Overload

11. _____ Principle of Progression

12. _____ Humidity

a) A method of training or physical conditioning in which a person moves through different exercises/stations in a timed manner. The primary purpose is to maintain an elevated HR while resistance training.

b) The stress applied must continually be perceived as new for the physiological system to adjust accordingly.

c) The period of time that an exercise session or training bout lasts.

d) The mechanics concerned with the effects force has on body motion.

e) An unconscious perception of movement and spatial orientation in relation to functional training controlled by specialized tissue and neural facilitation.

f) The amount of water vapor present in the air that affects the body's thermoregulation during exercise.

g) Exercises designed to develop muscular tone and promote physical fitness often used as a warm-up activity.

h) A training stress which challenges a physiological system of the body above the level which it is accustomed to.

i) Relatively small injuries in the body usually consisting of small tears in the muscle fibers.

j) The magnitude, or level of difficulty, in which an activity is performed, often expressed as a percentage of maximum.

k) For a desired adaptation to occur in the body a stress demand must be appropriately and specifically applied.

l) The number of times a person engages in a particular activity per given amount of time.

## Competency Exercises

1. List five ways that increasing muscle temperature will help improve efficiency and performance.

    1. _____

    2. _____

    3. _____

    4. _____

    5. _____


2. Give five beneficial reasons for implementing a cool down routine.

    1. _____

    2. _____

    3. _____

    4. _____

    5. _____


3. True or False? Cool downs should be employed following both moderate to high intensity anaerobic and aerobic exercise.


4. Provide four adaptational responses to the bodies physiology in response to routine aerobic exercise.

    1. _____

    2. _____

    3. _____

    4. _____


5. All of the following could be used as effective aerobic exercise modalities except:

    A. Swimming
    B. Jogging
    C. Power lifting
    D. Biking


6. True or False? If a client's goal is to compete in a running endurance event, his or her training regimen should include anaerobic training first, followed by aerobic training for each exercise bout.

7. Number, in order (1, 2, 3…8), the general training format when combining anaerobic and aerobic activities for a healthy adult with no underlying conditions.

_____Cool Down

_____Strength Training

_____Anaerobic Conditioning

_____Static Stretching

_____Aerobic Training

_____Dynamic Flexibility

_____Warm-up

_____Hypertrophy Training

8. Provide two reasons why recovery periods are necessary between successive bouts of exercise.

1. _____

2. _____

9. Name three program principles that are necessary components of an effective exercise routine.

1. _____

2. _____

3. _____

10. Provide five areas/conditions a trainer could monitor to improve a client's safety during the implementation of an exercise program.

1. _____

2. _____

3. _____

4. _____

5. _____

11. Describe five acute conditions specific to a client that, on any given day, a trainer should take into consideration prior to beginning any training.

1. _____

2. _____

3. _____

4. _____

5. _____

## Lesson Fifteen Quiz Questions

1. Exercise performance will shift from the anaerobic energy system and be replaced by the aerobic metabolism at about ____ minutes.

   A.  3
   B.  6
   C.  9
   D.  12

2. A 1:1 work to rest ratio is most commonly used for program sets in which of the following types of training?

   A.  Strength
   B.  Aerobic
   C.  Power
   D.  None of the above

3. Relative to training, the number of sets, repetitions, and training loads lifted is considered the training:

   A.  Intensity
   B.  Duration
   C.  Volume
   D.  Frequency

4. When considering progression, which of the following has the most rapid adaptation response?

   A.  Cardiovascular system
   B.  Metabolic system
   C.  Muscular system
   D.  Nervous system

5. As a general rule of thumb, progressive increases in exercise stress should be approximately _____ per week on average.

   A.  2-5%
   B.  6-9%
   C.  9-12%
   D.  13-15%

6. Which of the following is an example of overload?

   A.  Switching from bilateral to unilateral chest press on a physioball
   B.  Switching from weighted lunges to weighted lunges with trunk rotation using the same resistance
   C.  Switching from deadlift on a Smith machine to free weight deadlift using the same weight
   D.  All of the above

*Answers 1 A, 2 B, 3 C, 4 D, 5 A, 6 D*

## Lesson Sixteen
## Flexibility Assessment & Programming

### Learning Objectives

- Identify and discuss factors that may cause bilateral differences in ROM between joints
- List and discuss the benefits of flexibility training
- Identify problems and limitations associated with poor flexibility
- Explain how the different properties of flexibility affect range of motion
- Discuss the benefit of including myofascial release techniques in an exercise program
- List the factors that affect joint range of motion and explain how each may contribute to movement limitation
- Explain role of proprioceptors and mechanoreceptors in joint range of motion
- Identify the role of warm-up when designing a flexibility program
- List and define the different types of flexibility training
- Explain factors that determine flexibility technique selection and advantages and disadvantages of each
- Identify the prescription guidelines for static and dynamic flexibility training
- Perform flexibility training techniques and identify common errors in performance

## Match the Following Terms

1. _____Flexibility

2. _____Range of Motion (ROM)

3. _____Musculoskeletal

4. _____Fascia

5. _____Sarcomeres

6. _____Titin Filaments

7. _____Epimysium

8. _____Perimysium

9. _____Collagen

10. _____Mechanoreceptors

11. _____Osteophytes

12. _____Sacrum

a) Non-contractile protein filaments which make up the ends of the sarcomere.

b) The triangular bone made up of five fused vertebrae and forming the posterior section of the pelvis.

c) A fibrous tissue network enveloping, separating, or binding together muscles, organs, and other soft structures of the body.

d) The layer of connective tissue enveloping bundles of muscle fibers.

e) Small, abnormal bony growths.

f) The ability of a joint to move through a full range of motion.

g) The layer of connective tissue surrounding an entire muscle.

h) Relating to, or involving the muscles and the skeleton.

i) The fibrous protein constituent of bone, cartilage, tendon, and other connective tissue.

j) The achievable distance between the flexed position and the extended position of a joint that can be measured.

k) A segment into which a fibril of striated muscle is divided.

l) A specialized sensory end organ that responds to mechanical stimuli such as tension, pressure, or displacement.

## Fill in the Blanks with Appropriate Terms

1. _____ or joint laxity means a joint has an abnormal range of motion that compromises the joint's integrity due to reduced stability.

2. _____ is a technique used to correct fascia deformation and restriction using the application of rolling or static pressure on the tissue.

3. A form of stretching referred to as _____ usually involves a bouncing motion in which a limb or joint is forced into an extended range of motion using momentum, preventing the muscle from relaxing.

4. _____ is caused by stimulating the GTO via an increase of tension, creating an inhibitory effect on the muscle spindles.

5. _____ is a chronic autoimmune disease causing inflammation and deformity of the joints.

## Define the Following Terms

1. **Sarcopenia**:

2. **Bursitis**:

3. **Fasciitis**:

4. **Gout**:

5. **Proprioceptive neuromuscular facilitation (PNF)**:

6. **Dynamic flexibility**:

## Competency Exercises

1. Differences between bilateral joint movement capabilities are dependent upon several variables including:

    1. _____

    2. _____

    3. _____

    4. _____

2. List 5 benefits of flexibility.

    1. _____

    2. _____

    3. _____

    4. _____

    5. _____

3. When tight muscles compromise the kinetic chain affecting postural symmetry, it presents two main problems that promote joint injury. State the problem and negative effect it has on the body.

   First Problem: _____

_____

   Second Problem: _____

_____

4. Provide five functions the muscle's connective tissue serves.

    1. _____

    2. _____

    3. _____

    4. _____

    5. _____

5. List four functions that connective fascia serves in the body.

    1. _____

    2. _____

    3. _____

    4. _____

6. Name the three primary receptors used for neural management of the soft tissue related to ROM.

    1. _____

    2. _____

    3. _____

7. List five functions that articular mechanoreceptors perform to sense joint changes.

    1. _____

    2. _____

    3. _____

    4. _____

    5. _____

8. List the factors that, as one ages, may account for the functional diminution of muscle fibers.

    1. _____

    2. _____

    3. _____

    4. _____

9. True or False? Resistance training can aid in improving flexibility when performed correctly.

10. True or False? Bilateral movement seems to improve ROM better than uni-lateral movement.

11. Provide four common injuries related to ROM deficiencies.

    1. _____

    2. _____

    3. _____

    4. _____

12. Some specific elements commonly causing bursitis include:

1. _____

2. _____

3. _____

4. _____

5. _____

13. List three common causes of tendonitis.

1. _____

2. _____

3. _____

14. Name three of the most common diseases that can limit ROM.

1. _____

2. _____

3. _____

15. Provide four factors, other than aging, that may contribute to the development of Osteoarthritis.

1. _____

2. _____

3. _____

4. _____

16. True or False? During active stretching, the client being stretched supplies the force to lengthen the tissue.

17. A trainer should look at what key factors when determining which flexibility techniques should be incorporated into a training program?

1. _____

2. _____

3. _____

4. _____

18. True or False?  Static stretching performed at the beginning of a workout routine reduces force output.

## Lesson Sixteen Quiz Questions

1. _____ describes what causes the hamstring muscles to relax during quadriceps contraction.

   A.  Autogenic inhibition
   B.  Myofascial release
   C.  Reciprocal innervation
   D.  Hypermobility


2. Which activity would best serve to dynamically stretch the hip flexor?

   A.  Squat
   B.  Lunge
   C.  Step-up
   D.  Deadlift


3. Active-assisted stretching, proprioceptive neuromuscular facilitation, and active isolation all fall under the category of _____ flexibility.

   A.  Dynamic
   B.  Static
   C.  Ballistic
   D.  None of the above


4. _____ innervates the proprioceptors preventing muscle relaxation during the activity.

   A.  Ballistic stretching
   B.  Autogenic inhibition
   C.  Reciprocal innervation
   D.  Proprioceptive neuromuscular facilitation (PNF)


5. This type of flexibility is advantageous because it allows the body to gain flexibility from movements that can be employed before or during an exercise program.

   A.  Ballistic Stretching
   B.  Static Stretching
   C.  Dynamic Stretching
   D.  Proprioceptive neuromuscular facilitation (PNF)


*Answers 1 C, 2 B, 3 B, 4 A, 5 C*

# Lesson Seventeen
# Programming for Cardiovascular Fitness

## Learning Objectives

- Determine the appropriate cardiorespiratory test for varying populations
- Calculate predicted maximal heart rate and explain factors that affect the prediction
- Discuss the role of rate of perceived exertion and the "Talk Test" in programming for cardiorespiratory fitness
- Calculate target heart rate training zones using the Heart Rate Max Method and the Heart Rate Reserve Method and discuss relevant differences for exercise programming
- Identify recommended training intensities for varying populations
- Explain the differences between steady-state training and interval training for cardiorespiratory fitness
- Discuss the rationale for intensity selection and the advantages and disadvantages of high versus low intensity training
- Explain why the "fat-burning zone" may limit weight loss
- List the general guidelines for cardiorespiratory training
- Identify common expressions of energy expenditure
- Define a MET and explain its role in exercise programming
- Calculate energy expenditure using MET intensities
- Identify the relationship between energy expenditure and health
- List and discuss the different systems of training for cardiorespiratory fitness
- Discuss how genetics and age affect cardiorespiratory fitness
- Explain how exercise in the heat and at altitude affect cardiorespiratory training
- Identify how gender differences affect aerobic performance
- Explain the importance of recovery in cardiorespiratory exercise and how it differs from strength training
- Discuss methods to prevent a detraining effect
- Identify common injuries associated with cardiorespiratory exercise

## Match the Following Terms

1. _____Metronome

2. _____MET

3. _____Heart Rate Training Zone (HRTZ)

4. _____Graded Exercise Test (GXT)

5. _____Rate of Perceived Exertion (RPE)

6. _____Heart Rate Reserve (HRR)

7. _____Fartlek Training

8. _____Radiation

9. _____Convection

10. _____Conduction

11. _____Evaporation

12. _____Chondromalacia

13. _____IT Band Syndrome

14. _____Shin Splints

a) A type of interval training that uses steady-state pace with periodic variations in speed and grade.

b) The process in which heat is transferred from the body to a colder object upon contact.

c) An overuse injury, commonly associated with running, in which the iliotibial band becomes irritated due to the inflammation in the area.

d) The body's process of cooling, in which heat from the body is transferred into the air.

e) The process by which water is passed through the skin and is converted to water vapor, causing a cooling effect.

f) An instrument used to indicate the exact tempo at which work should be performed during certain tests (i.e., Step test).

g) A maximal aerobic test used to determine an individual's cardiovascular capacity.

h) The difference between heart rate maximum and resting heart rate (Max HR – Resting HR).

i) The metabolic equivalent of the oxygen consumed per minute while at rest.

j) One of the body's cooling methods in which heat from the body passes through the air into colder solids within close proximity.

k) The heart rate range that a person should work between in order to maximize his or her adaptation response to aerobic exercise.

l) Also known as medial tibial stress syndrome, the condition is commonly associated with overuse and is characterized by pain and tenderness over the middle or lower part of the shin bone.

m) A scale, usually numbered 6-20, that is used to monitor a client's own perception of his or her exertion during exercise.

n) Abnormal degeneration of the cartilage of the joints, especially in the knee, commonly associated with impact aerobic activities.

## Competency Exercises

1. List three potential problems that could create logistical issues related to maximal graded exercise tests (GXT).

1. _____

2. _____

3. _____

2. The classic formula to predict maximum heart rate is to subtract a person's _____ from 220.

    A. Resting HR
    B. MET level
    C. Age
    D. $VO_2$ at rest

3. A value of _____ on the RPE scale correlates with 60-80% of the heart rate reserve.

    A. 9-11
    B. 12-14
    C. 15-17
    D. 18-20

4. Research concludes that four factors may contribute to prediction error when using the traditional heart rate max formula including:

    1. _____

    2. _____

    3. _____

    4. _____

5. The equation for the Heart rate reserve (HRR) formula: _____ - Resting HR

    A. Maximum HR
    B. Percentage of $VO_2max$
    C. Age
    D. 200

6. What training goals suggest performing moderately intense training rather than high intensity training?

    1. _____

    2. _____

    3. _____

    4. _____

7. Fill in the following chart.

| Goal | Frequency | Duration |
|---|---|---|
| General Health | | |
| Fitness | | |
| Performance | | |

8. One liter (L) of oxygen used by the tissue equates to approximately _____ kcal burned.

    A. 3
    B. 5
    C. 8
    D. 9

9. A 154 lb. male sitting in a chair for 30 minutes consumes how many liters (L) of oxygen?

    A. 7.35 L
    B. 9.48 L
    C. 10.16 L
    D. 11.42 L

10. Provide the total caloric expenditure of a 264 lb. male exercising on an elliptical machine at 8 METS for 20 minutes.

    A. 236 kcal
    B. 274 kcal
    C. 336 kcal
    D. 396 kcal

11. List three factors that can modify the intensity during the different modes of aerobic training.

    1. _____

    2. _____

    3. _____

12. Provide three benefits of participating in a cross-training routine.

    1. _____

    2. _____

    3. _____

13. Improvement capabilities when participating in an aerobic exercise routine is dependent upon which four factors?

    1. _____

    2. _____

    3. _____

    4. _____

14. What four methods does the human body use to cool itself during exercise?

    1. _____

    2. _____

    3. _____

    4. _____

15. If training in environmentally heated conditions, which of the following is the body's primary mechanism to remove heat?

    A. Radiation
    B. Convection
    C. Conduction
    D. Evaporation

16. Explain the rationale (specifically the physiological adaptations) for athletes to perform their training at higher altitudes.

_____

_____

_____

17. Within the first few weeks of detraining, trained individuals show a decline in aerobic performance due primarily

to a reduction in _____ and consequent _____ diminution.

18. List five common injuries associated with aerobic training.

    1. _____

    2. _____

    3. _____

    4. _____

    5. _____

## Lesson Seventeen Quiz Questions

1. Which of the following describes the rationale behind the talk test?

   A. Defining an individual's maximum heart rate (MHR)
   B. Defining an individual's ventilatory threshold
   C. Defining an individual's heart rate reserve (HRR)
   D. Defining an individual's caloric expenditure

2. For proper cardiovascular improvements to take place, the training intensity for a deconditioned person starting an exercise program should be somewhere between which of the following training intensities?

   A. 30-40% Heart Rate Max
   B. 40-50% $VO_2$max
   C. 60-70% Heart Rate Reserve
   D. 70-80% Heart Rate Max

3. For proper cardiovascular improvements to take place, the training intensity for healthy individuals should be within which of the following heart rate max percentile zones?

   A. 55-70%
   B. 65-80%
   C. 75-90%
   D. None of the above

4. Which of the following would **not** be a factor when selecting the aerobic exercise intensity for a client?

   A. Current fitness level
   B. Exercise tolerance
   C. Muscle fiber distribution
   D. All of the above should be considered

5. A person with a $VO_2$max of 35 ml $\cdot$ kg$^{-1}$ $\cdot$ min$^{-1}$ has a maximal MET level of _____.

   A. 6
   B. 8
   C. 10
   D. 12

*Answers 1 B, 2 B, 3 C, 4 C, 5 C*

# Lesson Eighteen
# Anaerobic Training

## Learning Objectives

- List the benefits of resistance training and explain the physiological mechanism for each
- Explain the relationship between the anaerobic pathways and exercise programming
- Discuss how anaerobic testing is used in the development of a needs analysis
- List and define each of the resistance training systems and identify the role of each in exercise programming
- Discuss the difference between programming for muscular power, strength, hypertrophy, endurance, and fitness training and list the guidelines for each
- Identify the factors that determine recovery variations in different resistance training programs
- Explain the stretch-shortening cycle and its role in plyometric training
- Discuss the adaptation outcomes and challenges of concurrent anaerobic and aerobic training
- Compare and contrast adaptation responses to resistance training related to age and gender differences
- Explain how to reduce the effects of detraining during periods of reduced volume
- Identify common injuries associated with resistance training

---

## Fill in the Blanks with Appropriate Terms

1. The ratio of carbon dioxide produced by tissue metabolism to oxygen consumed in the same metabolism is known

   as the _____.

2. _____ is an insufficient supply of blood to a certain area of the body.

3. A hormone secreted by the pituitary gland called _____ is responsible for promoting bone and muscle growth in the body.

4. A hormone secreted by the testes called _____ is responsible for the development and maintenance of male secondary sex characteristics.

5. A stretching of the muscle into significant deformation or a tear of fibers due to excessive strain is referred to as a

   _____.

6. A stretching of the ligaments usually occurring when the joint becomes unstable during exertion or after a fall or sudden movement that violently pulls or twists the body is referred to as

   _____.

7. _____ is a condition in which there is a defect in the vertebra, usually the lower lumbar, typically caused by a stress fracture to the bone.

8. A condition marked by an instability between two involved vertebrae known as

   _____ is caused by genetic inheritance or a trauma to the upper of the two vertebrae.

9. _____ is an abnormal lateral curvature of the spine.

## Match the Following Terms

1. _____Priority System

2. _____Pyramid System

3. _____Superset System

4. _____Contrast System

5. _____Complex System

6. _____Drop Set System

7. _____Circuit System

8. _____Lactate Tolerance
        System

9. _____Negative Set System

a) A training approach based on the superset concept, used primarily for performance enhancement, emphasizing the combination of neuromuscular crossover between strength and power by performing a select number of repetitions to volitional failure followed by a similar exercise with less resistance at a faster speed.

b) A training approach usually comprised of 12-15 exercises where each exercise is performed for a predefined time period or repetition range before moving to the next exercise.

c) A training approach, particularly for new clients, that suggests performing exercises for deficient muscle groups first in an exercise bout.

d) A training approach which requires exercisers to lift a resistance that is greater than their 1RM, usually 105%-125% of maximum, by performing a controlled eccentric movement followed by a spot-assisted, concentric movement.

e) A training approach that utilizes the principle of neural preparation similar to a specific warm-up which requires exercisers to increase weight while decreasing repetitions in subsequent sets.

f) A training approach (also referred to as strip sets) that increases the demands on a particular muscle by using a set of repetitions to volitional failure before reducing the weight and performing the subsequent set without a rest interval.

g) A training approach in which the general concept is to perform one set of exercise immediately followed by a different exercise, with only transitional rest between sets.

h) A training approach in which a group of exercises are selected with a designated number of repetitions with a goal to complete all the repetitions of the exercises in the shortest period of time. The rest period is dependent upon the exerciser's ability to recover.

i) A training approach using a combination of agonist or agonist/antagonist exercises used in a grouping with varying rest periods.

## Competency Exercises

1. List five benefits of resistance training.

1. _____

2. _____

3. _____

4. _____

5. _____

2. True or False? Strength training enhances insulin sensitivity and improves both lean and adipose tissue

responsiveness to insulin.

3. Identify three activities that would require energy from the anaerobic phosphagen system in order to be successfully accomplished.

1. _____

2. _____

3. _____

4. Name the key factor in the glycolytic pathway that limits force production.

_____

5. Client-appropriate anaerobic endurance test selections should include which three considerations?

1. _____

2. _____

3. _____

6. Identify six key considerations a trainer must take into account when establishing an exercise program for a client.

1. _____

2. _____

3. _____

4. _____

5. _____

6. _____

7. Which of the following training approaches is commonly used for performance enhancement, emphasizing the combination of neuromuscular crossover between strength and power?

    A. Drop set system
    B. Lactate tolerance system
    C. Contrast system
    D. Circuit system

8. True or False? Exercises involving larger muscle groups will also benefit smaller muscle groups in hypertrophy training.

9. Ideally, hypertrophy training requires how much recovery time between training bouts of the same muscle group?

    A.  12-24 hours
    B.  24-36 hours
    C.  48-72 hours
    D.  None of the above

10. True or false? The nervous system is primarily responsible for strength gains obtained in the first three to five weeks of resistance training

11. List four common modes of training for power.

    1. _____

    2. _____

    3. _____

    4. _____

12. List five factors that have an effect on anaerobic endurance.

    1. _____

    2. _____

    3. _____

    4. _____

    5. _____

13. Explain the mechanism by which plyometric training has been shown to increase power output.

_____

_____

_____

14. Briefly explain how concurrent training, using both resistance and aerobic exercise, can have a negative and positive impact on each other.

_____

_____

_____

15. Provide three potential problems associated with velocity impairments in older adults.

    1. _____

    2. _____

    3. _____

16. List three physiological reasons for age-related decline in muscular strength, power, and size in older individuals.

    1. _____

    2. _____

    3. _____

17. True or False? Men and women alike demonstrate a similar ability to increase strength with age.

18. True or False? Findings suggest that most women can perform routine resistance training with little worry of increasing body segment circumference measures.

19. Explain how detraining due to cessation of resistive stress has a negative impact on muscle performance.

_____

_____

_____

20. The degree to which any of the myophysiological characteristics associated with resistive training cessation are affected is dependent upon which four factors?

    1. _____

    2. _____

    3. _____

    4. _____

21. List three possible hormonal changes that could occur as a result of detraining.

    1. _____

    2. _____

    3. _____


22. List four possible causes of muscle strains.

    1. _____

    2. _____

    3. _____

    4. _____


23. Provide the correct action for each letter of the acronym P.R.I.C.E in response to an acute injury.

    P- _____

    R- _____

    I- _____

    C- _____

    E- _____


24. Name the four muscles that make up the rotator cuff.

    1. _____

    2. _____

    3. _____

    4. _____

**Lesson Eighteen Quiz Questions**

1. Studies have shown that which of the following training programs helps prevent functional decline in the elderly?

   A.  Strength
   B.  Balance
   C.  Agility
   D.  Jump training
   E.  All of the above

2. Resistance training is important for obese individuals due to the effect it has on _____.

   A.  Reducing body fat
   B.  Preventing insulin resistance
   C.  Increasing aerobic fitness
   D.  All of the above

3. Which training system example would be best for hypertrophy training?

   A.  Back squat superset with box jumps
   B.  Chest press superset with push-ups
   C.  Shoulder press superset with calf raises
   D.  Bench press superset with bicep curls

4. _____ is the ideal training system for resistance training aimed at weight loss.

   A.  Pyramid system
   B.  Circuit system
   C.  Contrast system
   D.  Complex system

5. During bouts for maximal strength training, rest intervals of _____ minutes are necessary to fully rephosphorylate the phosphagen (ATP-CP) energy system.

   A.  <2
   B.  2-5
   C.  >5
   D.  None of the above

6. _____ is a training system that combines two or three different exercises without a rest interval.

   A.  Priority system
   B.  Circuit system
   C.  Superset system
   D.  Lactate tolerance system

7. A female begins a three-day a week exercise program, but does not want to perform resistance training for fear of gaining too much mass. Which of the following would be the correct response to encourage participation?

    A. Females have much lower testosterone levels making muscle growth difficult
    B. Females have much lower muscle hormone receptor concentration to testosterone produced in response to resistance training
    C. Resistance training for hypertrophy requires high volumes of training and relatively high intensity which can not be effectively accomplished training three times per week in females
    D. All are correct

8. Which of the following activities is commonly associated with rotator cuff injuries?

    A. Volleyball
    B. Baseball
    C. Tennis
    D. Swimming
    E. All of the above

*Answers 1 E, 2 B, 3 B, 4 B, 5 B, 6 C, 7 D, 8 E*

# Lesson Nineteen
# Resistance Training Technique

## Learning Objectives

- Compare and contrast the different types of strength training and explain the role of each in a resistance training program
- Explain the importance of skill acquisition when programming resistance training exercises
- Discuss proper breathing techniques during dynamic resistance training
- Explain how movement speed is determined when prescribing resistance training
- Discuss factors that affect program progressions in resistance training programs
- Implement correct spotting techniques for resistance training exercise
- Discuss the role hand position plays in exercise performance and modification
- Calculate resistance training intensity based on repetition performance using the 3% formula
- Identify the relationship between repetition range and training intensity
- Implement proper resistance training techniques and identify common errors

---

## Match the Following Terms

1. _____ Manual resistance

2. _____ Free weight

3. _____ Ergonomics

4. _____ Rhomboids

5. _____ Central Nervous System

6. _____ Latissimus dorsi

7. _____ Biceps brachii

8. _____ Triceps brachii

9. _____ Lordosis

10. _____ Timed-Intensity Technique

a) Broad, triangular shaped muscles connecting from the vertebral column to the humerus, responsible for shoulder extension and humeral adduction.

b) An abnormal increase in the natural curvature of the spine in the lumbar region.

c) The science of equipment set-up intended for maximal work efficiency and safety.

d) Consists of the brain, spinal cord, and connecting nerves.

e) A resistance training technique in which the trainer applies resistance to the movement of an exercise.

f) A lifting technique using a time-to-failure strategy to designate a proper weight.

g) Rhombus-shaped muscles of the back that are chiefly responsible for scapular retraction.

h) A muscle of the upper arm (posterior) mainly responsible for extending the elbow.

i) Resistance that has no attachment to a machine with the resistive force provided by the gravitational pull on the object.

j) A muscle of the upper arm (anterior) mainly responsible for flexing the elbow.

## Competency Exercises

1. Briefly explain why doing a push-up from the floor is much more difficult than performing the same exercise with hands on an elevated bench.

_____

_____

_____

2. Briefly explain the technique of manual resistance.

_____

_____

_____

3. Name three positive adaptations encouraged when using the whole body during resistive training (i.e., weighted squats).

    1. _____

    2. _____

    3. _____

4. Explain a possible advantage of using machines instead of free weight and body weight movements.

_____

_____

_____

5. Explain some of the disadvantages of using machine resistance training.

_____

_____

_____

6. True or False? Controlled breathing is a fundamental part of proper movement execution during resistance lifting.

7. Explain why the use of proper progressions in resistance training is vital to successfully programming the CNS for desired movement patterns and advancing adaptations.

_____

_____

_____


8. List three challenges one can use to progress an exercise program.

    1. _____

    2. _____

    3. _____


9. Identify the three different types of hand positions generally used during resistance training exercise.

    1. _____

    2. _____

    3. _____


10. Explain why different hand positions might be selected when participating in free weight resistive training.

_____

_____

_____


11. True or False? When spotting deadlift exercises, a trainer should place one hand on the low back of the client with the other supporting the chest.

## Lesson Nineteen Quiz Questions

1. Older adults and beginning exercisers are often initially steered toward which type of training, reducing the transfer benefit of resistance training into functional improvement.

   A. Free weight training
   B. Body weight training
   C. Resistance machine training
   D. Stability equipment

2. Which specific client population in particular should closely regulate their breathing technique to adequately manage internal pressure during resistance exercise?

   A. Hypertensive clients
   B. Adolescent clients
   C. Elderly clients
   D. A & C only
   E. None of the above

3. The use of slower, controlled speeds during resistive exercises increases the duration of time stress is placed on the muscle, thereby increasing _____.

   A. Muscle fiber recruitment
   B. Risk for muscle fiber tears
   C. Muscle fiber atrophy
   D. All of the above

4. When supine presses are performed with a dumbbell, where should the trainer spot the exercise?

   A. Hands on or near the weight
   B. Hands on or near the distal end of the forearm
   C. Hands on or near the elbow
   D. Hands on or near the distal end of the humerus

5. How should a trainer spot a lifter performing a Back Squat?

   A. Stand behind the lifter, placing their hands on or near the client's rib cage just under the chest
   B. Stand behind the lifter, placing one hand on the low back and one on the sternum
   C. Stand behind the lifter, placing hands on the client's hips
   D. Stand behind the lifter, placing hands on or near the bar
   E. All of the above are acceptable

6. What percentage of a 1RM should a client generally do when performing 10-12 repetitions of an exercise?

   A. 60-65%
   B. 70-75%
   C. 80-85%
   D. 90-95%

*Answers 1 C, 2 D, 3 A, 4 B, 5 A, 6 B*

# Lesson Twenty
# Functional Training Concepts

## Learning Objectives

- Define functional training and explain its role in health attainment
- Explain the concept of proprioception and how it affects exercise performance
- Compare and contrast traditional resistance training and functional training
- Identify the role of stability in functional training and discuss methods used to challenge it in exercise progressions
- Demonstrate how traditional exercises can be modified into functional exercises
- Identify variables used in exercise progressions for functional training
- List and discuss programming considerations when implementing functional-based training
- Discuss general program recommendations for functional training
- Perform functional exercises and identify common errors

## Match the Following Terms

1. _____ Functional training

2. _____ Motor learning

3. _____ Synergist

4. _____ Pectoralis major

5. _____ Anterior deltoid

6. _____ Axial skeleton

7. _____ Appendicular musculature

a) The muscle of the anterior part of the shoulder connecting from the anterior border of the clavicle to the lateral aspect of the humerus.

b) The name given to a muscle which assists in performing the same joint movement as the agonist.

c) The primary musculature of the arms and legs.

d) Training targeted at enhancing coordinated movements specifically designed at improving function in activities necessary for everyday living.

e) A series of sequential phases (cognitive, associative, and autonomous) involved in learning to perform a movement task in response to a given stimulus.

f) The large muscle connecting the anterior aspect of the chest with the shoulder and upper arm.

g) The bones of the skeleton including the skull, spinal column, sternum, and rib cage.

## Competency Exercises

1. Briefly explain the difference between traditional and functional training.

_____

_____

_____

2. True or False? The different resistance modalities used in function-based training do not require force production for increased muscular strength.

3. Explain why a standing military press often necessitates less resistance than the seated military press.

_____

_____

_____

4. Explain why a strong core foundation is essential when performing functional training.

_____

_____

_____

_____

5. Provide three potential, subsequent problems that result from a lack of neuromuscular coordination.

    1. _____ which can lead to,

    2. _____ which can lead to,

    3. _____

6. List four ways to exercise selection can help enhance proprioception.

    1. _____

    2. _____

    3. _____

    4. _____

7. Provide an example of how the functionality of exercise may be altered for each of the following exercises.

| Exercise | Example Altered Exercise |
| --- | --- |
| Push-up on the floor | _____ |
| Forward lunge | _____ |
| Bench press | _____ |
| Leg curls | _____ |
| Side lateral raise | _____ |

8. True or False? If neuromuscular coordination and balance is the goal, traditional formats including intensity and set-repetition schemes should be emphasized over functional exercises.

9. List two ways in which the intensity of a throwing activity can be adjusted to elicit a wide variety of force couples in the trunk and appendicular musculature.

1. _____

2. _____

10. Different pieces of exercise equipment are designed to enhance functionality by moving the body from a

_____, _____,

into less stable _____.

11. List five different pieces of exercise equipment commonly used to enhance functionality in an exercise routine.

1. _____

2. _____

3. _____

4. _____

5. _____

## Lesson Twenty Quiz Questions

1. The unconscious perception of spatial orientation, movement, and muscular tension is known as:

   A. Mental alertness
   B. Functional surrounding
   C. Proprioception
   D. Motor learning

2. Which of the following resistance modalities are least likely to enhance performance stability?

   A. Resistance machines
   B. Free weight resistance
   C. Functional resistance
   D. None of the above

3. The number of sets and repetitions used in functional training are based on which of the following factors?

   A. Client specificity
   B. Goal specificity
   C. Exercise specificity
   D. All of the above

4. Functional training emphasizes actions aimed at:

   A. Force production
   B. Hypertrophy
   C. Endurance proficiency
   D. Movement efficiency

5. Which of the following would be an example of a function-based exercise?

   A. Dumbbell bench press
   B. Romanian deadlift
   C. Asymmetrically loaded step-up
   D. Single-arm seated row
   E. All of the above

*Answers 1 C, 2 A, 3 D, 4 D, 5 C*

# Lesson Twenty One
# Creating and Exercise Program

## Learning Objectives

- Identify the steps used to enhance exercise program design
- Explain how the needs analysis defines program goals and activity selection
- Discuss the FITT principle and explain why it has limitations in exercise programming for personal training
- Identify the stages of program development starting with a needs analysis
- Identify the main factor which defines the method of exercise modification
- Discuss the rationale for program cycles and explain how periodization plays a role in ongoing adaptation response
- Explain the role of program tracking and how it is used for program evaluation and risk management

## Competency Exercises

1. List four factors specific to personal training that contribute to the challenges of exercise programming.

   1. _____

   2. _____

   3. _____

   4. _____


2. Personal trainer programs are designed to cater to each individual client by identifying and managing what four general areas?

   1. _____

   2. _____

   3. _____

   4. _____


3. In the creation of a needs analysis, what issues are paramount in a training program when priority ranking has identified a need for the client?

   1. _____

   2. _____

   3. _____

4. A traditional training approach to exercise programming uses the FITT principle. Identify what each letter stands for in the acronym FITT.

  F- _____

  I- _____

  T- _____

  T- _____

5. True or False? Aerobic exercise is not necessarily beneficial for overall improved health and the reduction of disease compared to resistance training.

6. Briefly explain why energy system considerations will dictate the order of the program components in a training bout.

_____

_____

_____

7. True or False? Sport-specific training differs from general health and fitness training as the emphasis is on the performance components of fitness.

8. Why should a client with a reduced physical capacity have a program with higher repetitions incorporated into his/her exercise routine?

_____

_____

_____

9. Identify three successive problems with administering progressions too aggressively in a workout routine.

  1. _____

  2. _____

  3. _____

10. A key consideration when implementing a workout routine is that the body adapts to stress based on what three concepts?

    1. _____

    2. _____

    3. _____

11. True or False? The number of times a client engages in the program components will determine the rate of adaptation and subsequent progression.

12. List five different components of exercise that can be modified to refine the program stress delivery.

    1. _____

    2. _____

    3. _____

    4. _____

    5. _____

13. An actual training cycle length will be based upon which four considerations?

    1. _____

    2. _____

    3. _____

    4. _____

14. Briefly explain the rationale behind segmenting a training routine.

_____

_____

_____

15. True or False? In periodization, the concept is to accomplish one group of adaptations to support the next.

16. The traditional periodization approach uses a four stage preparation phase including what four phases?

1. _____      Phase

2. _____      Phase

3. _____      Phase

4. _____      Phase

## Lesson Twenty One Quiz Questions

1. In personal training, an effort should be made to combine exercises whenever possible in order to:

   A.  Save time
   B.  Increase training volume
   C.  Increase performance demands
   D.  All of the above

2. Which of the following is a prescription priority in an exercise routine designed for an individual with high blood pressure?

   A.  Resistance exercise
   B.  Aerobic exercise
   C.  Plyometric training
   D.  Flexibility training

3. For individuals with limited mobility, progressions in exercise should focus on which of the following?

   A.  Increased movement range
   B.  Increasing MET intensity
   C.  Linear force production
   D.  All of the above

4. Why should fitness testing results and evaluative criteria be incorporated into an exercise program?

   A.  To create foundations for prescribed stress
   B.  To ensure each defined objective is appropriately met
   C.  To monitor and assess training effectiveness
   D.  All of the above

5. In most cases, training cycles can last _____ weeks:

   A.  6
   B.  8
   C.  10
   D.  12
   E.  All of the above may be correct

*Answers 1 D, 2 B, 3 A, 4 D, 5 E*

## Lesson Twenty Two
## Working with Special Populations

### Learning Objectives

- Explain the etiology of asthma and identify signs and symptoms and common triggers that may cause an episode
- Discuss how physical activity affects the asthmatic condition and risks associated with exercise
- List general recommendations for exercising with asthma
- Determine modifications of the exercise program to allow for safe participation for individuals with asthma
- Identify emergency procedures in the event of an asthma attack
- Discuss the differences between type I and type II diabetes
- Explain the etiology of type II diabetes and lifestyle factors that contribute to its development
- List the benefits of exercise on the diabetic condition
- Explain how the different types of exercise affect diabetes
- List the general recommendations for exercise for type I and type II diabetes
- Identify general concerns and recommendations to avoid hyperglycemia and hypoglycemia for individuals exercising with diabetes
- List the benefits of exercise for pregnant females and the unborn child
- Discuss the physiological adjustments that occur with pregnancy
- Identify general recommendations for exercise during pregnancy and activities that should be avoided
- List the contraindications for exercise during pregnancy
- Identify blood pressure values associated with hypertension
- Explain the role exercise plays in managing hypertension
- Identify specific concerns related to resistance training and hypertension and strategies to implement anaerobic exercise in a personal training program
- List the general recommendations and guidelines for exercise and hypertension
- Explain the role of exercise in CAD and its effect on atherosclerotic reversal
- List the general recommendations for exercise and CAD
- Prescribe different modes of exercise for individuals with CAD
- Discuss the etiology of Congestive Heart Failure
- Identify concerns and limitations related to CHF and exercise
- Explain modifications required for exercise for individuals with CHF
- List the general recommendations for exercise and CHF
- Identify the benefits of exercise for children
- Explain the physiological differences between children and adults in response to exercise
- Discuss concerns and limitations for children participating in exercise
- List the general guidelines for children and exercise
- Identify the importance of exercise by mode and intensity for older adults
- List the benefits of exercise for older adults
- Discuss considerations for exercise and older adults
- Prescribe exercise modifications for older adults

## Match the Following Terms

1. _____ Exercise induced asthma (EIA)
2. _____ Tidal volume
3. _____ Retinopathy
4. _____ Nephropathy
5. _____ Peripheral neuropathy
6. _____ Residual volume
7. _____ Pre-eclampsia
8. _____ Fibrinolysis
9. _____ Atherosclerosis
10. _____ Angina
11. _____ Congestive heart failure (CHF)
12. _____ Sleep apnea
13. _____ Thermoregulation

a) The volume of air remaining in the lungs after a maximal expiratory effort.

b) Chest pain or discomfort often resulting from restricted blood flow to the heart.

c) The process of actively maintaining a constant internal body temperature regardless of the surrounding environment.

d) An abnormal state of pregnancy in which there are signs of elevated blood pressure, water retention, and protein excretion in the urine.

e) A medical condition characterized by shortness of breath induced by exercise.

f) A small vessel disease or damage to the nerves predominantly in the arms and legs.

g) The volume of air inspired or expired in a single breath during regular activity.

h) The build-up of plaque on the inside of the blood vessels.

i) A non-inflammatory disease of the retina.

j) A condition caused by the heart's inability to maintain adequate blood circulation in the peripheral tissues and the lungs, marked by a significant reduction in stroke volume, reduced valvular function, and shortness of breath.

k) A condition in which breathing is interrupted or even stops periodically during sleep.

l) A disease or abnormality of the kidneys.

m) The process where a fibrin clot (blood clot), the product of coagulation, is broken down.

## Competency Exercises

1. List six preventative strategies to avoid asthma attacks when exercising.

1. _____
2. _____
3. _____
4. _____
5. _____
6. _____

2. List three improvements older adults may experience by engaging in routine aerobic exercise.

    1. _____

    2. _____

    3. _____


3. What can a trainer do to help prevent the incidence of Exercise Inducted Asthma (EIA) when implementing exercise strategies?

    1. _____

    2. _____

    3. _____


4. Type II diabetes is caused by several mechanisms including:

    1. _____

    2. _____

    3. _____

    4. _____


5. List three positive adaptations of a combined aerobic and resistance exercise circuit on a diabetic individual.

    1. _____

    2. _____

    3. _____


6. Name seven benefits pregnant women may gain from engaging in a moderate-intensity exercise program.

    1. _____

    2. _____

    3. _____

    4. _____

    5. _____

    6. _____

    7. _____

7. True or False? It is recommended that pregnant women should participate in exercise programs at moderate, submaximal levels based on individual criteria and with physician approval.

8. True or False? Pregnant exercisers should not perform resistance exercise routines.

9. List three physiological changes experienced during pregnancy that possibly increase the risk of injury when exercising.

   1. _____

   2. _____

   3. _____

10. For clients with CVD, trainers should note that different participation levels will be based on several disease-related factors including:

    1. _____

    2. _____

    3. _____

    4. _____

11. Identify four damaging effects to the body associated with hypertension (high blood pressure).

    1. _____

    2. _____

    3. _____

    4. _____

12. True or False? With hypertensive populations, exercise training at moderate intensities does not appear to lower blood pressure as much as exercise at higher intensities.

13. List four risk factors attributed to coronary artery disease (CAD) that can be affected by exercise.

    1. _____

    2. _____

    3. _____

    4. _____

14. Provide three cardiovascular benefits of participation in regular aerobic exercise for clients with CAD.

    1. _____

    2. _____

    3. _____

15. Briefly explain how resistance training combined with endurance training can significantly benefit clients with coronary artery disease (CAD).

_____

_____

_____

16. The level of appropriate exercise participation for individuals with coronary artery disease is based upon what three factors?

    1. _____

    2. _____

    3. _____

17. Exercise prescription for clients with CAD should be managed and monitored to determine lifting loads and movements by factoring in four criteria including:

    1. _____

    2. _____

    3. _____

    4. _____

18. Briefly explain how resistance training modalities should be structured differently for clients with congestive heart failure (CHF).

_____

_____

_____

_____

_____

19. When compared to adults, children are more efficient in terms of achieving steady-state heart rates during aerobic activities, due to which three factors?

1. _____

2. _____

3. _____


20. True or False? When training children, lower repetition (6-8) and higher weight schemes provide greater benefits compared to higher repetition (13-15), lower weight schemes.

**Lesson Twenty Two Quiz Questions**

1. The participation in resistance training activities is recommended for individuals with diabetes to:

    A. Improve blood glucose levels and insulin resistance
    B. Reduce HDL cholesterol
    C. Increased cardiac output
    D. All of the above

2. What is the possible consequence of a client with diabetes taking insulin immediately prior to an exercise bout?

    A. Hyperglycemia
    B. Hypoglycemia
    C. Hypertension
    D. Angina

3. What is the most common medical complication trainers should be aware of when training a pregnant client?

    A. Hypertension
    B. Cardiac disorders
    C. Gestational diabetes mellitus (GDM)
    D. Muscle dystrophy

4. Which of the following activities should be avoided when training pregnant clients?

    A. Aerobic training at 70% heart rate max intensity after the second trimester
    B. Supine crunches after the first trimester
    C. Resistance training after the first trimester
    D. All of the above

5. Which is the **least** important component to aerobic exercise programming used for a hypertensive client?

    A. Intensity
    B. Frequency
    C. Modality
    D. Total daily work completed

6. Which of the following should be regarded with the **most** concern when training a hypertensive client?

    A. Heavy Resistance training
    B. Moderate Aerobic training
    C. Flexibility training
    D. Functional exercises

7. Prior to engaging in resistance training, individuals with CAD should do which of the following?

    A. Be medically screened and cleared
    B. Be able to perform body weight exercise
    C. Perform aerobic exercise for at least 4 weeks
    D. All of the above

8. When training a client with CHF, which of the following methods would best be used in gauging exercise intensity?

   A. Heart rate
   B. RPE
   C. Blood Pressure
   D. Time

9. Which of the following physiological differences account for lower stroke volumes in children compared to adults?

   A. Heart size
   B. Blood vessel size
   C. Muscle mass
   D. Lung capacity

10. The primary physiological difference affecting the thermoregulation of heat between children and adults is related to:

   A. Fat distribution patterns
   B. Blood volumes
   C. Sweating mechanisms
   D. Heart size

11. Which of the following demonstrates both the greatest capacity to assess functional decline and substantially improve function in the elderly?

   A. Resistance exercise
   B. Aerobic exercise
   C. Flexibility training
   D. None of the above

12. Similar to children, training major muscle groups in elderly clients _____ times per week, at a moderate intensity, is sufficient for physiological improvements.

   A. 1 to 2
   B. 3 to 4
   C. 4 to 5
   D. 6 to 7

*Answers 1 A, 2 B, 3 C, 4 B, 5 C, 6 A, 7 A, 8 B, 9 A, 10 C, 11 A, 12 A*

# Lesson Twenty Three
# Ethics and Professional Behavior

## Learning Objectives

- Identify behaviors and actions that contribute to professionalism
- Discuss the professional principles and how they contribute to professionalism
- Discuss common standards of the personal training profession
- List and explain the components of the professional decision-making process
- Explain the components of risk management and identify strategies to reduce risk for liability
- Explain the importance of liability insurance for the personal trainer
- Identify steps to reduce the impact of a risk management occurrence
- List factors that contribute to an effective risk management plan

---

## Competency Exercises

1. Defined professional standards are useful in providing guidance for which of the following?

   A. Professional behaviors
   B. Overall decision-making processes
   C. Activities used
   D. Providing the framework for self-evaluation
   E. All of the above


2. Which of the following would **not** be considered a common standard of the personal training profession?

   A. Validly assessed and documented attainment of the minimal competency standards
   B. Proper representation of one's academic achievement, skills, and abilities
   C. Maintaining appropriate files and documenting all professional activity
   D. The referral of clients to the appropriate health care practitioners
   E. None of the above


3. Put the appropriate number next to each successive step in a professional decision-making process (i.e. 1, 2, 3…).

   _____Develop alternatives (Establish criteria, consider all the aspects…)

   _____Analyze the outcome (Learn from your actions)

   _____Implement the solution (Premeditate a plan, properly communicate…)

   _____Gather information (Collect facts/data; differentiate opinion & assumptions…)

   _____Record the findings (Use for future decision-making)

   _____Select the best course of action (Rank by appropriateness, suitability…)

   _____Identify the problem (Is it a goal, challenge, or opportunity?)

   _____Monitor the effect (Analyze the process or the result…)

   _____Weigh the alternatives (Identify advantages/disadvantages, benefits/consequences)

4. A legitimate credential/certification should uphold three requirements in regards to the specific testing procedures.

    1. _____

    2. _____

    3. _____

5. The ethical foundation in a client/professional relationship is built on which three ideas?

    1. _____

    2. _____

    3. _____

6. True or False? When a trainer receives anything of substantial value, including royalties, from companies in the health industry such as a manufacturer of supplements and fitness devices, this fact is required by law to be disclosed to clients or colleagues.

7. Name three general categories of potential risk that a personal trainer should be aware of. Give an example and a viable preventative plan for each example.

    1. Potential risk: _____

       Example: _____

       Preventative action: _____

       _____

    2. Potential risk: _____

       Example: _____

       Preventative action: _____

       _____

    3. Potential risk: _____

       Example: _____

       Preventative action: _____

       _____

8. Identify the six subsequent steps of risk management.

    1. _____

    2. _____

    3. _____

    4. _____

    5. _____

    6. _____

| | | | |
|---|---|---|---|
| Trapezius | Occipital-T12 | Scapula, Acromion process, Clavicle | Elevation, Upward rotation, Retraction, Depression (lower) |
| Rhomboids | C7-T5 | Scapula | Retraction, downward rotation |
| Teres Major | Inferior scapula | Medial humerus | Extension, medial rotation, and adduction |
| Biceps | Coracoid Process (short head), Scapula (long head) | Radius | Flexion of elbow (both heads), Supination of forearm (long head) |

| **Seated Calf Raise** | **Origin** | **Insertion** | **Action** |
|---|---|---|---|
| Soleus | Posterior tibia and fibula | Calcaneus | Plantar flexion |

| **Step-Ups** | **Origin** | **Insertion** | **Action** |
|---|---|---|---|
| Gluteus Maximus | Posterior sacrum and ilium | Distal lateral femur | Hip extension |
| Vastus Lateralis | Posterior femur, greater trochanter of femur | Patella and tibial tuberosity | Knee extension |
| Vastus Medialis | Posterior femur | Patella and tibial tuberosity | Knee extension |
| Vastus Intermedius | Anterior and lateral femur | Patella and tibial tuberosity | Knee extension |
| Rectus Femoris | Long head: Anterior inferior iliac spine<br>Short head: acetabulum | Patella and tibial tuberosity | Knee extension, Hip flexion |
| Semitendonosus | Ischial tuberosity | Anterior proximal tibia | Extension of hip, Flexion and medial rotation of flexed knee |
| Semimembranosus | Ischial tuberosity | Anterior proximal tibia | Extension of hip, Flexion of knee and medial rotation of flexed knee |
| Bicep Femoris | Long head: Ischial tuberosity<br>Short head: Posterior femur | Head of fibula | Long head: extension of hip<br>Both heads: flexion of knee |
| Gastrocnemius | Medial head: Medial epicondyle of femur<br>Lateral head: Lateral epicondyle of femur | Calcaneus | Plantar flexion, Knee flexion |

| **Traditional Dead lift** | **Origin** | **Insertion** | **Action** |
|---|---|---|---|
| Gluteus Maximus | Posterior sacrum and ilium | Distal lateral femur | Hip extension |
| Vastus Lateralis | Posterior femur, greater trochanter of femur | Patella and tibial tuberosity | Knee extension |
| Vastus Medialis | Posterior femur | Patella and tibial tuberosity | Knee extension |
| Vastus Intermedius | Anterior and lateral femur | Patella and tibial tuberosity | Knee extension |
| Rectus Femoris | Long head: Anterior inferior iliac spine<br>Short head: acetabulum | Patella and tibial tuberosity | Knee extension, Hip flexion |
| Semitendonosus | Ischial tuberosity | Anterior proximal tibia | Extension of hip, Flexion and medial rotation of flexed knee |
| Semimembranosus | Ischial tuberosity | Anterior proximal tibia | Extension of hip, Flexion of knee and medial rotation of flexed knee |
| Bicep Femoris | Long head: Ischial tuberosity<br>Short head: Posterior femur | Head of fibula | Long head: extension of hip<br>Both heads: flexion of knee |
| Gastrocnemius | Medial head: Medial epicondyle of femur<br>Lateral head: Lateral epicondyle of femur | Calcaneus | Plantar flexion, Knee flexion |

| Romanian Dead lift | Origin | Insertion | Action |
|---|---|---|---|
| Gluteus Maximus | Posterior sacrum and ilium | Distal lateral femur | Hip extension |
| Vastus Lateralis | Posterior femur, greater trochanter of femur | Patella and tibial tuberosity | Knee extension |
| Vastus Medialis | Posterior femur | Patella and tibial tuberosity | Knee extension |
| Vastus Intermedius | Anterior and lateral femur | Patella and tibial tuberosity | Knee extension |
| Rectus Femoris | Long head: Anterior inferior iliac spine<br>Short head: acetabulum | Patella and tibial tuberosity | Knee extension, Hip flexion |
| Semitendonosus | Ischial tuberosity | Anterior proximal tibia | Extension of hip, Flexion and medial rotation of flexed knee |
| Semimembranosus | Ischial tuberosity | Anterior proximal tibia | Extension of hip, Flexion of knee and medial rotation of flexed knee |
| Bicep Femoris | Long head: Ischial tuberosity<br>Short head: Posterior femur | Head of fibula | Long head: extension of hip<br>Both heads: flexion of knee |
| Gastrocnemius | Medial head: Medial epicondyle of femur<br>Lateral head: Lateral epicondyle of femur | Calcaneus | Plantar flexion, Knee flexion |

Medical clearance                    1

Hypertension 100 - Diastolic
160 - Systolic
    if 140/90 - workout w/ caution
        leg press - impacts blood pressure

> 135 - LDL cholesterol
< 40 HDL good cholesterol

Total > 220                waist cir : 40 males
Ratio LDL/HDL  5:1                    35 Females

RHR = 100

Body fat % = W 40%
                M 30%

BMI = overweight - 25
        obese 30
    35 Femal
    40 males